W9-APB-039

American Medical Association

Guide to
Living with Diabetes

American Medical Association

Guide to
Living with Diabetes

Preventing and Treating Type 2 Diabetes—
Essential Information You and Your
Family Need to Know

American Medical Association

Boyd E. Metzger, M.D.

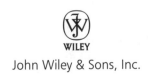

WILEY

John Wiley & Sons, Inc.

Copyright © 2006 by the American Medical Association. All rights reserved

Published by John Wiley & Sons, Inc., Hoboken, New Jersey
Published simultaneously in Canada

Design and composition by Navta Associates, Inc.

Credits: Bar graph on insulin sensitivity adapted from the work of Richard N. Bergman, Ph.D: 11; National Eye Institute, National Institutes of Health: 184; © PhotoDisc: 72, 177; Think-stock/PunchStock: 116 (right); USDA photos by Ken Hammond: 116 (left), 198, 225, and 244.

The recommendations and information in this book are appropriate in most cases and current as of the date of publication. For more specific information about a medical condition, the AMA suggests that you consult a physician.

For general information about our other products and services, please contact our Customer Care Department within the United States at (800) 762-2974, outside the United States at (317) 572-3993 or fax (317) 572-4002.

Wiley also publishes its books in a variety of electronic formats. Some content that appears in print may not be available in electronic books. For more information about Wiley products, visit our web site at www.wiley.com.

Library of Congress Cataloging-in-Publication Data:

The American Medical Association guide to living with diabetes : essential information you and your family need to know about preventing and treating type 2 diabetes / American Medical Association.
    p. cm
  Includes index.
  ISBN-13 978-0-471-75023-9 (cloth)
  ISBN-10 0-471-75023-9 (cloth)
  1. Non insulin-dependent diabetes—Popular works. I. American Medical Association.
  RC662.18.A44 2006
  616.4'62—dc22

                              2006005496

Printed in the United States of America

10 9 8 7 6 5 4 3 2

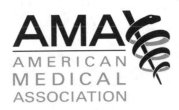

Michael D. Maves, MD, MBA   *Executive Vice President, Chief Executive Officer*

Bernard L. Hengesbaugh   *Chief Operating Officer*

Robert A. Musacchio, PhD   *Senior Vice President, Publishing and Business Services*

Anthony J. Frankos   *Vice President, Business Products*

Mary Lou White   *Executive Director, Editorial and Operations*

Boyd E. Metzger, MD   *Medical Editor*

Donna Kotulak   *Managing Editor/Writer*

Pam Brick   *Writer*

Mary Ann Albanese   *Art Editor*

Contents

Introduction

More than 19 million Americans have diabetes—a condition that can produce life-threatening complications. Of the two major forms of diabetes—type 1 and type 2—type 2 comprises 90 to 95 percent of all cases in the United States. An additional 13 million people have the precursor to type 2 diabetes, called prediabetes. Worldwide, type 2 diabetes affects more than 190 million people, and some experts predict that if the current trends continue that figure could surge to over 300 million by the year 2025.

Diabetes is one of the leading causes of death and disability in the United States, and annual diabetes-related medical costs total more than $100 billion. The predicted future increase in the number of cases is fueled by several factors. Americans are becoming increasingly sedentary and overweight; being overweight is the major risk factor for type 2 diabetes. Age is another factor—most cases of type 2 diabetes develop after age 45. In addition, Hispanic Americans and other minority groups who have a high incidence of type 2 diabetes make up the fastest-growing segment of the US population.

The good news is that type 2 diabetes can often be prevented, mainly by eating a healthy and balanced diet, getting regular exercise, and keeping your weight within a healthy range. If you are overweight, losing just 5 to 7 percent of your weight (that's 10 to 14 pounds if you weigh 200 pounds) and keeping it off can cut your risk in half.

If you already have diabetes, close monitoring of your blood sugar levels along with healthy eating and regular exercise can help you manage your condition and avoid serious complications. Even small changes in your lifestyle can produce big health benefits. This book is designed to help you learn how to make those changes in your daily life that can help you avoid type 2 diabetes or, if you have type 2 diabetes, maintain good control of it and reduce your risk of complications.

PART ONE

Type 2 Diabetes: A Modern Epidemic

1

What Is Diabetes?

D iabetes is a medical disorder that affects the way the body uses food for growth and energy. When you eat, the carbohydrates (starches and sugars) are broken down into glucose, a simple sugar that is one of the main sources of fuel for your body. As food is digested, glucose gets absorbed into the bloodstream, which transports it throughout the body. Muscle and fat cells respond to signals from a circulating hormone in the blood called insulin, which is the "key" that unlocks the "doors" of these cells to enable glucose to enter and do its work. People who have diabetes either don't have enough insulin or their cells have become insensitive, or resistant, to the effects of insulin. As a result, glucose doesn't get into the cells and it begins to build up in the blood. This buildup of glucose in the blood is the hallmark of diabetes.

Previously known as adult-onset or non-insulin-dependent diabetes, type 2 diabetes used to develop almost exclusively in people who were over age 40 and overweight. Over the past decade, however, the number of children and young adults diagnosed with type 2 diabetes in the United States has climbed dramatically because of the growing epidemic of obesity that often begins in childhood.

The high blood sugar concentration brought on by both forms of diabetes can cause serious long-term complications such as nerve damage, heart disease, kidney failure, blindness, and amputation.

An uncontrolled blood sugar level can also cause severe short-term complications such as loss of consciousness, and can even be fatal. Many people with type 2 diabetes can control their blood sugar with diet, exercise, and weight loss, but some need to take sugar-lowering medications or insulin injections.

Type I Diabetes

Although the major concern of this book is type 2 diabetes, which is far more common than type 1 diabetes, it is helpful to understand the difference between the two forms. People with type 1 diabetes completely lose the ability to produce the hormone insulin. The specialized beta cells in the pancreas stop generating enough insulin to keep blood sugar levels normal. This type of diabetes can begin at any age but is most

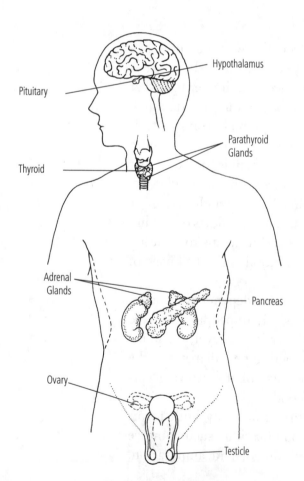

Pituitary

Hypothalamus

Thyroid

Parathyroid Glands

Adrenal Glands

Pancreas

Ovary

Testicle

The Endocrine System

The endocrine system is a group of glands and tissues shown here that secrete hormones into the bloodstream to coordinate and control many essential body processes. The pancreas is the organ most involved in diabetes because its most important job is to regulate blood sugar (glucose) levels. The pancreas produces the hormones insulin and glucagon (which regulate the body's use of glucose, fats, and proteins). The pancreas also secretes digestive enzymes that help break down food and convert it into glucose. The pituitary is the "master gland" that makes hormones that control several other endocrine glands. The hypothalamus, just above the pituitary gland in the brain, controls hormone secretion by the pituitary and is the main link between the endocrine and nervous systems. The thyroid gland produces the hormones thyroxine and triiodothyronine, which control the rate at which cells burn fuel for energy. The four parathyroid glands release parathyroid hormone, which helps regulate the level of calcium in the blood. The adrenal glands produce hormones including corticosteroids (which influence metabolism and the body's response to stress) and epinephrine, or adrenaline (which increases blood pressure and heart rate during times of stress). The ovaries produce the female hormones estrogen and progesterone; the testicles produce male hormones (androgens, primarily testosterone).

often diagnosed in young people. The peak time of onset is between ages 8 and 18.

Type 1 diabetes is an autoimmune disorder in which the immune system mistakenly identifies specific body tissues—in this case the beta cells of the pancreas—as foreign and attacks and destroys them. The precise cause of this error in immune function is unknown, but experts think that some people are born with a genetic susceptibility to it. Then, at some point in their life, an environmental trigger such as a virus or a toxin activates this genetic susceptibility to bring on the errant immune response that produces type 1 diabetes.

The symptoms of type 1 diabetes tend to come on quickly and severely, unlike those of type 2 diabetes, which often remain unnoticeable over a period of several years. Symptoms of type 1 diabetes include weakness, weight loss, excessive hunger and thirst, blurred vision, and increased urine output.

People with type 1 diabetes reach the point at which they do not produce enough insulin to survive, so for the rest of their lives they must take regular doses of insulin, usually by injection under the skin. Insulin cannot be taken by mouth because digestive enzymes would destroy it before it could reach the bloodstream.

Type 2 Diabetes

People who have type 2 diabetes make insulin, but their cells do not respond to it in the normal way. The body's resistance, or lack of sensitivity, to the effects of insulin characterizes type 2 diabetes, formerly known as adult-onset or non-insulin-dependent diabetes. Many factors can cause people to have insulin resistance, but being overweight and physically inactive and eating an unhealthy diet are among the most important. In the United States, 85 to 90 percent of people with type 2 diabetes are overweight or obese (more than 20 percent over their ideal body weight).

Type 2 diabetes usually develops after age 40. However, with the surge in obesity in the United States and around the world, the age at which this form of diabetes is diagnosed is dropping. Today, very overweight children and young adults are developing type 2 diabetes at rates unheard of just a decade ago. (See chapter 14 to learn more about children and type 2 diabetes.)

What Is Type 2 Diabetes?

Type 2 diabetes is a medical disorder in which the body has difficulty using insulin to control the level of the sugar glucose in the blood. When type 2 diabetes first develops, the pancreas still produces a lot of insulin but not enough to maintain the normal processing of glucose in muscles, fat, and the liver. This decreased ability to process glucose eventually causes it to build up in the blood, leading to diabetes.

The early stages of type 2 diabetes, which often last several years, produce no symptoms. But even without noticeable symptoms, high

The Role of Blood Sugar

To be healthy, your body needs to keep its blood sugar (glucose) level within a narrow range: between 70 and 110 milligrams per deciliter (mg/dL) of blood, measured when you have not eaten for several hours or overnight. The blood glucose level rises after eating, but in healthy people it seldom rises above 150 or 160 mg/dL after meals. Doctors generally measure blood sugar levels after a person has fasted because sugar levels can remain above the fasting level for several hours after eating.

The pancreas is one of the key organs that maintains blood sugar levels within normal limits. The pancreas is located across the midsection of the body just behind the lower part of the stomach. The pancreas performs a number of important functions. For example, it secretes digestive juices that contain enzymes to break down food into particles, or molecules, tiny enough to be absorbed and used by cells. But perhaps the most important job of the pancreas is to make insulin, a hormone that controls the way muscle and fat cells use and store sugar.

After you eat, your intestines break down and absorb the carbohydrates (or sugars) in the food and release them into the liver and the bloodstream, which carries the sugars throughout the body so that your cells can use them for energy. As the level of sugar, or glucose, rises in your blood, the pancreas quickly begins to churn out insulin, which stimulates muscle and fat cells to take up excess glucose from the blood. These tissues store the surplus glucose until your body needs it, bringing the blood glucose level back into the normal range.

The pancreas also produces a hormone called glucagon, which has the opposite effect of insulin. When the glucose in your blood starts to get too low—such as when you haven't eaten in a while or during vigorous exercise—the pancreas secretes glucagon to prevent the glucose level from falling too low. Glucagon signals the liver and muscle cells to release the glucose they have stored into the bloodstream to allow the blood sugar level to rise. Glucagon also stimulates the liver to produce glucose out of protein found in the body.

In these ways, glucagon keeps the blood sugar level from dropping too low and causing symptoms of hypoglycemia (which can include sudden hunger, dizziness, shakiness, nervousness, irritability, confusion, and drowsiness). Severe hypoglycemia, which can lead to seizures and lack of consciousness, requires emergency medical treatment. When functioning normally, this delicate balance between insulin and glucagon precisely regulates the sugar level in the blood, keeping it within the healthy range.

glucose levels can damage nerves and blood vessels and cause complications such as heart disease, kidney failure, stroke, and blindness. Initially, the pancreas keeps blood sugar normal by releasing more and more insulin. But when insulin output starts to decline, blood sugar begins to go up. Eventually, the pancreas becomes exhausted—its output of insulin falls progressively and the amount of glucose in the blood continues to rise, while muscle and fat cells are starved of the energy they need. Over time, this situation can lead to symptoms such as thirst, weight loss, frequent urination, and lack of energy similar to the symptoms of type 1 diabetes.

However, this intricate system can become disrupted under certain stresses, such as obesity, especially when fat is concentrated around the abdominal area. If your cells are resistant to the effects of insulin, your body needs more insulin to maintain normal blood glucose levels. If your body cannot increase its output of insulin sufficiently, your muscle and fat cells can't use glucose fully and the liver starts making more glucose. Blood glucose then increases and can eventually lead to type 2 diabetes. Elevated blood glucose is the hallmark of diabetes.

How the Body Processes Glucose

The pancreas and the liver are the two major organs that help control glucose levels in the blood. Glucose, which is absorbed from digested food into the intestines, is the sugar that cells in the body use for energy. The pancreas secretes two hormones, insulin and glucagon, that have opposite effects in response to blood glucose levels: insulin lowers blood glucose and glucagon raises blood glucose. When blood glucose is high, the pancreas secretes insulin to stimulate liver, fat, and muscle cells to take in glucose from the bloodstream. When blood glucose is low, the pancreas secretes glucagon to stimulate the liver to release stored glucose into the bloodstream and to increase the rate at which the liver makes glucose.

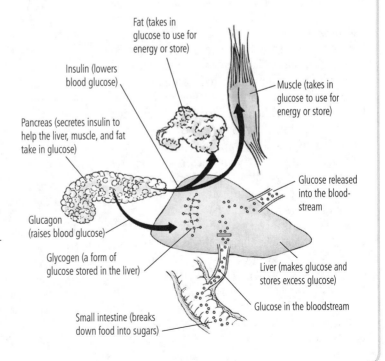

Fat (takes in glucose to use for energy or store)

Insulin (lowers blood glucose)

Muscle (takes in glucose to use for energy or store)

Pancreas (secretes insulin to help the liver, muscle, and fat take in glucose)

Glucose released into the bloodstream

Glucagon (raises blood glucose)

Glycogen (a form of glucose stored in the liver)

Liver (makes glucose and stores excess glucose)

Glucose in the bloodstream

Small intestine (breaks down food into sugars)

How Insulin Works

Insulin is a hormone secreted by an organ called the pancreas. Inside the pancreas are several hundred thousand clusters of cells called islets. One type of islet cell, the beta cell, secretes insulin in response to the rise in glucose in the bloodstream. Like all hormones, insulin circulates in the bloodstream and can affect the function of cells, organs, and tissues throughout the body. The muscle and fat cells in your body have receptors on their surfaces to which insulin can attach as it circulates in the blood. Once insulin attaches itself to a receptor on the surface of a cell, the cell switches on other functions in the cell that attract and absorb glucose into the cell from the blood. The cell then converts the glucose into energy or stores it for future use.

If your pancreas does not make enough insulin, your muscle cells cannot take in sufficient amounts of glucose for your body's energy needs. Without insulin, your fat cells release their stored energy too fast. The excess fat gets broken down in the liver to form chemicals called ketone bodies, which can build up in the blood and cause a life-threatening condition called ketoacidosis. Ketoacidosis can lead to diabetic coma or even death. You can eat normal amounts of food but lose weight or even become malnourished because your body is not properly processing the food. This can occur if the pancreas is unable to produce insulin, as in type 1 diabetes, or if your cells have become resistant to the effects of insulin and your pancreas cannot keep up with the increased demand for insulin, as in type 2 diabetes.

Insulin was discovered in 1921 in Canada, and the first insulin preparations for treating diabetes were developed in 1922. The discovery of insulin was a major step forward in diabetes treatment. Before the availability of insulin, people with type 1 diabetes died within months to a few years of their diagnosis. The early insulin preparations were derived from the pancreases of cows and pigs. Although these insulin preparations treated type 1 diabetes successfully in most affected people, some people had adverse reactions to impurities in the insulin preparations. By the 1980s, scientists had discovered how to make human insulin in large quantities by inserting copies of the human gene for insulin production into bacteria and manipulating the bacteria to make insulin.

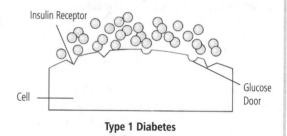

Type 1 Diabetes

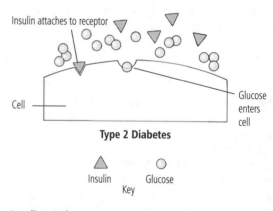

Type 2 Diabetes

Insulin's Role

Insulin is a hormone that enables muscle and fat cells to take in glucose (sugar) from the blood to use for energy or store for future energy needs. In a person with type 1 diabetes, the pancreas has stopped producing insulin; without insulin, the cells—even though they have receptors ("keys") for insulin and "doors" to let in glucose—do not take in glucose. In a person with type 2 diabetes, the cells have become unresponsive to insulin; although insulin attaches to the receptors, glucose has difficulty entering the cells. In both forms of diabetes, glucose builds up in the bloodstream—quickly in type 1 diabetes and gradually in type 2 diabetes.

How Type 2 Diabetes Develops

Type 2 diabetes is a disorder that has two major components: insulin resistance (when the body is less sensitive or responsive to the hormone insulin) and reduced ability of the pancreas to make and secrete a sufficient amount of insulin to keep blood glucose at a normal level. Among healthy people, there is a broad range in sensitivity to insulin, and a person's sensitivity to insulin can fluctuate at different stages of life and still keep glucose levels within the healthy range. For example, whites tend to be more sensitive to insulin than Mexican Americans. Older people and people who are overweight or obese tend to be less sensitive to insulin than children and people who are thin or at a healthy weight. Insulin sensitivity tends to decrease during puberty and during the second and third trimesters of pregnancy. These are all normal ranges of insulin sensitivity in healthy people—their pancreas increases its output of insulin as the muscle and fat cells become less sensitive to the effects of insulin and the level of glucose in their blood remains normal.

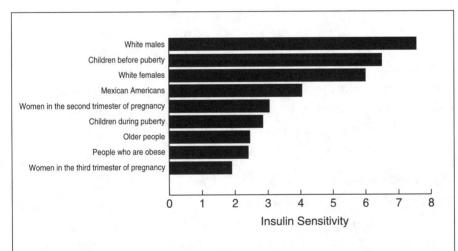

Normal Variations of Insulin Sensitivity

The chart here shows normal variations in insulin sensitivity among healthy people. Most hormones are required in similar amounts in everyone and have similar effects on them, but insulin is different. Healthy people can vary greatly in how responsive their body is to the effects of insulin; problems develop only when blood glucose cannot be kept at a normal level.

Some people (such as whites) are more sensitive to insulin than others (such as Mexican Americans), and this sensitivity can fluctuate throughout life but still effectively maintain blood glucose within the healthy range. Increasing age and being obese can make the body less sensitive to insulin, and insulin sensitivity tends to decrease during puberty and the later stages of pregnancy.

However, if the function of the insulin-producing beta cells in the pancreas is impaired and the increased insulin output by the pancreas no longer sufficiently matches the decreased insulin sensitivity, glucose begins to build up in the blood. In the next phase, as glucose continues to build up in the blood, symptoms of type 2 diabetes eventually develop, along with related metabolic changes (such as abnormalities in cholesterol and other blood fats).

Insulin Resistance

If you have insulin resistance, your body's cells are not responding as well—are less sensitive or more resistant—to the effects of the hormone insulin. Insulin resistance is a key factor in the development of type 2 diabetes. At the level of the cell, insulin connects to an insulin receptor on the cell surface that normally triggers a specific communication pathway inside the cell, relaying signals telling the cell to perform certain functions. For reasons that are not fully understood, these cellular signals fail to function normally, blocking the cell's ability to respond to the signals from insulin. Normally, insulin signals muscle and fat cells to take in the sugar glucose for energy. The disruption in this communication pathway often results from the presence of excess fats in the bloodstream resulting from the effects of insulin resistance in fat cells and the liver.

When the cells are no longer sensitive to the effects of insulin, the pancreas compensates by producing more and more insulin, up to twice or even three times the normal rate. Researchers are trying to understand what triggers this increased production of insulin.

What Causes Insulin Resistance?

Obesity and lack of activity are thought to be the major causes of insulin resistance, although other environmental factors as well as genes also play a role. Age is also a factor: insulin sensitivity tends to decrease with age. Excess stress can cause cell-damaging inflammation, which increases insulin resistance. Hormones play a role by acting directly or indirectly on muscle or fat cells to increase their resistance to insulin. This may partly explain why women tend to become less sensitive to insulin after menopause, when their body produces less estrogen and other female hormones. Women become insulin resistant when they are pregnant (see page 243). In rare cases, insulin resistance can be brought on by a medication or by some medical conditions (such as Cushing's disease, which results from an excess of corticosteroid hormones in the blood).

The Consequences of Insulin Resistance

If you eat more calories than your body burns, you store the excess energy as fat throughout your body. Some people store a higher proportion of fat in and around their abdomen and less around their hips and thighs. When excess fat is concentrated in the abdominal area (producing a "beer belly" and an apple shape) rather than generalized under the skin throughout the body and around the hips (producing "love handles" and a pear shape), a person is more likely to be insulin resistant. Abdominal fat also makes a person more likely to have abnormal blood fats (dyslipidemia)—an increase in potentially harmful fats in the blood called triglycerides and a decrease in beneficial high-density lipoprotein (HDL) cholesterol.

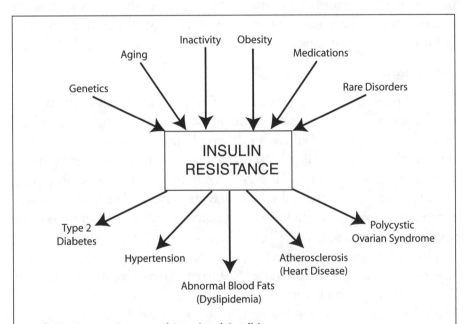

Insulin Resistance: Causes and Associated Conditions

Insulin resistance is influenced by a number of factors, both environmental and genetic. The two most important risk factors are obesity and lack of activity. But age, family history, and ethnicity are also important. Less commonly, insulin resistance is brought on by a medication or a rare medical disorder. Insulin resistance in turn can accompany or worsen a number of conditions that often occur together. If you are insulin resistant, you are more likely than people who are not insulin resistant to have diabetes, hypertension, abnormal cholesterol levels, heart disease, or polycystic ovarian syndrome.

As fat cells get filled with stored triglycerides, they become less and less able to respond to insulin, and they start discharging fatty acids into the bloodstream. These fats released by the cells quickly end up circulating in the bloodstream as triglycerides and other potentially damaging fatty acids, increasing insulin resistance and setting the stage for heart disease.

In addition to dyslipidemia, insulin resistance is associated with several other conditions, including type 2 diabetes, polycystic ovarian syndrome (see page 29), high blood pressure (see page 93), and atherosclerosis (see page 166).

Some people who have insulin resistance and a high level of insulin in their blood, primarily children and young adults, develop dark patches of skin on the back of their neck, on their elbows, knees, or knuckles, or in their armpits; some may have a dark ring around their neck. This condition is called acanthosis nigricans (see page 207). People who develop acanthosis nigricans may have a higher risk of going on to develop type 2 diabetes than people who are equally insulin resistant but do not have acanthosis nigricans.

Prediabetes

Before a person's blood glucose levels have reached levels high enough to be considered type 2 diabetes, he or she usually enters a stage called prediabetes, characterized by borderline high glucose levels. Without intervention such as major lifestyle changes or glucose-lowering medication, a person with prediabetes is likely to go on to develop type 2 diabetes and is at increased risk of having a heart attack or a stroke. From a diagnosis of prediabetes to the onset of type 2 diabetes takes an average of eight years.

Doctors diagnose prediabetes by the presence of impaired fasting glucose or impaired glucose tolerance (see page 28), two conditions that can be identified by blood tests. Ten to 15 percent of adults in the United States have either impaired fasting glucose or impaired glucose tolerance.

Impaired fasting glucose and impaired glucose tolerance, often referred to together as prediabetes, are part of the continuum that can lead to type 2 diabetes. But having prediabetes does not mean that going on to type 2 diabetes is inevitable. Many people with prediabetes can take measures to delay or prevent type 2 diabetes. The most important goals of these measures are to prevent blood sugar from rising any further and, in the best of all situations, to lower blood sugar to a healthy level. Doctors recommend that people at this stage work hard to lose 5 to 7 percent of their body weight and exercise regularly for at least 30 minutes every day.

A healthy diet (see chapter 4) is an essential part of preventing type 2 diabetes. You will need to make major changes in your eating habits to improve both the quality and the quantity of food you eat. Your doctor or dietitian can help you develop a dietary plan that supplies all your nutritional needs and fits your lifestyle. Generally, a healthy diet is low in fat and calories; provides carbohydrates, proteins, and fats in percentages recommended by your doctor or dietitian; and is rich in fiber. It includes plenty of fruits, vegetables, whole grains, and legumes, along with fish (at least two or three times a week), which provides heart-healthy omega-3 fatty acids.

In research studies, a medication called metformin has been shown to be effective in treating impaired fasting glucose and impaired glucose tolerance and can help halt the progression to type 2 diabetes. However, metformin doesn't work as well in lowering glucose as lifestyle changes do. If your doctor has told you that you have impaired fasting glucose or impaired glucose tolerance, your first goal should be to make the extra effort to eat more healthfully and exercise to lose weight.

Doctors can detect impaired fasting glucose and impaired glucose tolerance using the following tests:

Fasting Blood Glucose Test The fasting blood glucose test is usually done first thing in the morning and measures blood sugar after a person has gone without eating for 10 to 14 hours (usually overnight). Fasting glucose levels of 100 to 125 mg/dL are above normal but not high enough to indicate a diagnosis of diabetes. Instead, these levels indicate impaired fasting glucose (IFG) or prediabetes.

Glucose Tolerance Test The glucose tolerance test is done after a 10- to 14-hour fast. Blood is taken after a person has fasted and again 2 hours after he or she drinks a sweet liquid provided by the doctor's office. Blood sugar levels between 140 and 199 mg/dL measured 2 hours after drinking the liquid are considered above normal but are not high enough to indicate a diagnosis of diabetes. These levels indicate impaired glucose tolerance (IGT). Like impaired fasting glucose, it indicates an increased risk of developing type 2 diabetes.

If you are 45 years old or older, are at a normal weight, and don't have a family history of type 2 diabetes, your doctor will probably test you for prediabetes and related conditions every three years, even if you don't have any other risk factors for type 2 diabetes (see chapter 2). If you have insulin resistance syndrome (see box on page 13) or any of the associated conditions, you may be tested at a younger age and more frequently. This is also true if you have ever developed diabetes during a pregnancy (see chapter 15).

Consider an unfavorable test result your motivator to make beneficial lifestyle changes—such as losing weight and becoming more physically active. Physical activity and weight loss make your cells more sensitive to insulin. Many people with prediabetes are able to bring their blood sugar down sufficiently to enable their body to use insulin effectively again, reducing their risk of developing type 2 diabetes and its potential complications.

Insulin Resistance Syndrome

If a person has prediabetes, he or she is likely to also have one or more of the following conditions because they often occur in people who have insulin resistance and prediabetes.

- Obesity (especially when concentrated around the abdomen)
- High levels of triglycerides in the blood (150 mg/dL or higher)
- Low levels of beneficial HDL cholesterol (under 40 mg/dL in men and under 50 mg/dL in women)
- High blood pressure (130/85 mm Hg or higher)
- Polycystic ovary syndrome (see page 29), a condition that usually (but not always) affects obese women

Individually, these conditions increase the risk of cardiovascular (heart and blood vessel) disease and type 2 diabetes; having three or more increases the risk even more. If you have three or more of these conditions, you have what doctors refer to as insulin resistance syndrome.

Because of the cardiovascular and diabetes risks linked to insulin resistance syndrome, if you have prediabetes (have been diagnosed with impaired glucose tolerance or impaired fasting glucose), your doctor may want to determine if you have other features of insulin resistance syndrome. If you do have other features, your doctor will recommend treatment for each of them. For example, if you have high blood pressure, your doctor will recommend lifestyle changes (such as exercise and weight loss) and may prescribe an antihypertensive medication to bring your blood pressure down to a healthy level. For high cholesterol, your doctor will also recommend lifestyle changes and possibly a cholesterol-lowering medication. If you are overweight, your doctor will recommend a weight-loss strategy.

Treating each of these conditions will help reduce your cardiovascular risks (including heart disease, heart attack, and stroke). Lifestyle changes—eating better, losing weight, and exercising more—will also help reduce your insulin resistance and your risk of developing type 2 diabetes.

Keep in mind that none of these conditions—high blood pressure, abnormal cholesterol levels, or elevated glucose levels—has symptoms at the early stages; you can have any of them for several years and not know it. That's why it is so important to have a complete physical examination and blood tests regularly—especially if you are overweight and have a family history of type 2 diabetes. You should also talk to your doctor about testing for your child if your child is obese and you have a family history of diabetes. (See chapter 14 to learn more about children and type 2 diabetes.)

Why Is Type 2 Diabetes on the Rise?

The incidence of type 2 diabetes has jumped 50 percent in the last 10 years, and the number of people with type 2 diabetes in 2025 is predicted to be more than double the number in 1995. Experts warn that if current trends continue, one in three people born in the year 2000 will develop the disorder during his or her lifetime. What factors are causing this steep rise in type 2 diabetes? The short answer is that people, both adults and children, are eating too much, exercising too little, and getting fatter.

Overeating and a sedentary lifestyle work together to cause obesity. But the regular consumption of high-calorie foods isn't the whole story. Obesity is a complicated condition that results from a dynamic mix of genetic, psychological, and socioeconomic factors. In some cases, obesity can result from a medical condition or a medication. Gender also plays a role. Women burn fewer calories at rest than men because they have less muscle mass (muscle burns more calories than fat). As we age, we tend to lose muscle, and then fat accounts for a higher percentage of our weight. Metabolism also slows with age, so our body requires fewer calories. If you don't eat fewer calories or exercise more as you age, you will lose muscle, put on fat, and gain weight over time—and that excess weight puts you at risk for type 2 diabetes.

Being inactive promotes obesity because fewer calories are burned at rest. This may seem obvious, but many people never think about how active, or inactive, they are. Having a desk job, driving to work, watching TV, and surfing the Internet take up a large portion of most Americans' day. But the human body was designed for movement and, without it, starts to break down and have problems, like a car that isn't used for years. Overall fitness and health require regular physical activity. Obesity and lack of exercise make muscle and fat cells less sensitive to insulin. When a person is both overweight and sedentary, this effect is multiplied.

2

Are You at Risk?

Many of the same factors that put you at risk for insulin resistance syndrome also increase your risk of developing type 2 diabetes. These risks include inherited factors, such as family history and ethnicity, and lifestyle factors such as obesity, inactivity, a poor diet, and smoking.

But even if you have inherited genes or have family traits that make you susceptible to developing type 2 diabetes, it does not mean that you are destined to develop it. Lifestyle factors have a strong influence on whether you will develop type 2 diabetes. The disorder tends to be triggered by environmental stresses such as being overweight and inactive. Even people with the diabetes susceptibility genes can significantly reduce their risk of diabetes by eating a healthy diet, keeping their weight within a normal range, and being physically active.

Obesity

Being overweight is a very important risk factor for type 2 diabetes. The vast majority of people with type 2 diabetes are overweight. The more you weigh, the higher your risk for type 2 diabetes. Obesity, which doctors define as being more than 20 percent over your ideal weight, is the fastest-growing health problem in the United States. The number of

How to Measure Your Waist

Your waist size is a gauge of your future health risks because it is an indication of how much fat is deposited in and around your abdomen. Even if your weight is in the normal range, your risk of developing health problems such as type 2 diabetes and heart disease is increased if you tend to gain weight in your abdominal area. If you are a man whose waist measures more than 40 inches or a woman whose waist measures more than 35 inches—that is, your abdominal area is larger around than your hips and thighs—your risk of diabetes and heart disease is further increased.

To properly measure your waist, locate your upper hipbone. Place a measuring tape around your abdomen just above the top of the hipbone, keeping the measuring tape parallel to the floor and snug around your waist, but don't pull it so tightly that it pulls in your waist. Relax and read the measurement as you exhale. If you are not sure whether you have measured your waist properly, ask your doctor to measure it at your next checkup.

Americans who are obese is 75 percent higher than in the early 1990s, and it continues to increase. During the same period, the incidence of type 2 diabetes rose 61 percent. The coinciding increase in obesity and type 2 diabetes is striking evidence of their close relationship.

Calculating body mass index (BMI; see page 35) is also a way to diagnose obesity. A BMI of above 27 in men and above 25 in women indicates overweight. Generally, the higher your BMI, the higher your risk of having health problems such as heart disease, high blood pressure, and type 2 diabetes.

Obesity can be especially harmful if you carry more weight in your abdomen than on your hips and thighs—even if your BMI is less than 27—because fat inside the abdomen makes the cells less sensitive to insulin, which regulates blood glucose. This lack of sensitivity, or resistance, to the effects of insulin is an important factor in the development of type 2 diabetes. When abdominal fat is high, the function of the insulin-producing beta cells in the pancreas tends to be impaired and the level of fat in the blood (in the form of triglycerides) is likely to increase. These effects make glucose even more difficult to regulate. These and other health risks are substantially increased in men whose waist measures 40 inches or more and in women whose waist measures 35 inches or more.

Age

Although the incidence of type 2 diabetes is increasing among obese children and young adults, it is still most common after age 45. For reasons that are unclear, the functioning of the insulin-producing beta cells of the pancreas tends to decrease as people age. There is also a tendency for the cells of older people to be less sensitive to insulin. Without a sufficient supply of insulin in the blood to regulate glucose, the risk of type 2 diabetes increases.

Family History

Your family health history is a key factor to consider when evaluating your risk for type 2 diabetes. If one of your parents or a sibling has type 2 diabetes, your chances of developing the disease are much higher than people in families with no diabetes. Although there is a genetic component in type 2 diabetes, it does not mean that type 2 diabetes is simply an inherited disorder. Doctors think that the interaction of several genes and environmental factors have the most impact on a person's susceptibility to type 2 diabetes.

For example, Native Americans have the highest incidence of type 2 diabetes in the world. But a hundred years ago, the disease was rare among Native Americans. One group, the Pimas of Arizona, has an incidence of type 2 diabetes that is several times higher than that of whites of European descent, while their genetic cousins, the Pimas living in rural Mexico, have a low incidence of type 2 diabetes. What is it in the lives of Native Americans during the last century that could have produced this stunning reversal? What accounts for the disparity between the diabetes rates of the Pimas of Arizona and the Pimas of Mexico? Because the Pima groups are so similar genetically, the answer must lie with differences in their lifestyle and environment.

The Arizona Pimas switched to the typical American diet that is high in fat, salt, sugar, and calories, and their physical activity declined sharply. As a result, they became obese and their diabetes rate skyrocketed. Even though the Mexican Pimas have the same genes, their diabetes rates remain very low because they eat a high-fiber diet with lots of whole grains and fresh fruits and vegetables and they engage in strenuous physical activity.

Most Americans don't exercise enough. These lifestyle factors—eating too much and exercising too little—appear to adversely affect, or "switch on," the genes of people who are susceptible to developing type 2 diabetes. Regardless of the way the genetic vulnerability works, people with a family history of type 2 diabetes need to be especially conscientious when it comes to eating a nutritious diet, getting regular exercise, and keeping their weight down.

If you are not sure if anyone in your family has had type 2 diabetes, ask your parents, aunts and uncles, and grandparents if they know of any close family members with the disorder.

Ethnicity

People in some ethnic groups have a higher risk for type 2 diabetes than others. In North America, for example, diabetes is more of a threat to Native Americans, African Americans, Hispanics, Asians, Pacific Islanders, and Native Alaskans than it is to people of northern European descent. In Australia, diabetes affects the native (indigenous) population in greater numbers than it does other groups. The reasons for this discrepancy are still unclear, but researchers see some interesting links between ethnicity and what they think are "thrifty genes."

Compared with the diet of our ancestors, our diet differs in many ways. Not only does it contain more fat, sugar, salt, preservatives, and other food additives, but much of our food is also processed and refined. During the processing of foods, some of the food's nutrients may be lost. Another big difference is that food is available and easy to obtain at any time of the day or year. All we have to do is reach into the cupboard or the refrigerator and, when we run out of something, drive to the grocery store to stock up on more. And if we don't feel like going to the grocery store, we can order our groceries online and have them delivered to our door. If we don't feel like cooking, we can eat at a restaurant and order from a menu of diverse meal choices that are likely to contain deep-fried, high-fat, and other calorie-dense foods in enormous portions. Desserts, snacks, and treats are ever-present. Food advertising floods our senses from the TV, radio, billboards, and magazines. Some researchers think that these two major differences—the abundance and easy availability of food and the minimal amount of exercise required today to obtain food—are major factors in the dramatic increase in type 2 diabetes.

The theory of thrifty genes suggests that humans have genes that allow fat to be easily stored by the body when food is plentiful to have available for use later, when food is scarce or in times of famine. Having these genes was a great advantage to people who went through frequent periods of food shortages caused by environmental threats such as drought. But today, when we have an abundant food supply all the time and limited need for physical activity to perform our daily routine, these genes can be a problem because we don't burn the excess fat our body efficiently stores. In other words, the human body has not had time to adapt to this new lifestyle—and the result, for many of us, is obesity, insulin resistance, and type 2 diabetes.

Lifestyle Factors

Like most people, you probably feel pulled between the demands of your job and your family. When you are busy, you may be less inclined to eat right and exercise. An unhealthy diet and a lack of exercise can increase your chances of getting type 2 diabetes because they tend to lead to weight gain. Maybe you smoke cigarettes or drink alcohol to excess to relieve stress. Smoking-induced illnesses are the number one preventable cause of death in the United States. Smoking increases your risk of serious health problems, including unfavorable cholesterol levels, cardiovascular disease, high blood pressure, stroke, and type 2 diabetes. Excessive drinking can increase your heart risks by raising blood pressure and the level of potentially harmful triglycerides (fats) in the blood.

An Unhealthy Diet

Our hectic lifestyle has led many of us to shortchange ourselves when it comes to eating a healthy diet. Many Americans are consuming foods containing too many unhealthy saturated and trans fats (see page 50) and too much sugar and salt. One of the biggest reasons for this trend is our affection for fast foods, which are generally high in unhealthy fats, calories, and salt.

Fast Foods

The consumption of fast foods has risen dramatically in the United States in recent decades and is now responsible for more than a third of all restaurant food expenditures. A 4-ounce hamburger with cheese and all the trimmings supplies 700 to 800 calories, 30 grams of fat, plus 1,100 milligrams of sodium (about half the recommended daily sodium allowance). French fries provide an additional 200 to 500 calories (depending on serving size), 40 percent of which come from fat.

Although some fast-food restaurants are now cooking their fries in healthier vegetable oils, many still deep-fry them in potentially harmful partially hydrogenated oils, which are trans fats. Trans fats are especially unhealthy because they increase the level of LDL (the "bad" cholesterol in the blood) more than other types of dietary fat. Trans fats are present in a wide variety of foods on grocery shelves, including cookies, snack crackers, potato and tortilla chips, doughnuts, pastries, cakes, and pies. These foods are high in calories and provide few other nutrients. Trans fats are sometimes contained in foods you would not expect to find them in, such as some breakfast cereals, breads, and broths—so read food labels carefully when shopping. Watch for the terms "hydrogenated oil," "partially hydrogenated oil," and "trans fats" on food labels and ingredient lists on packaged foods and avoid those that contain them.

Saturated Fat

A high intake of saturated fat, present in fatty red meat, the skin of poultry, and cheese and other full-fat dairy products, has long been known to contribute to high levels of cholesterol and other blood fats. Although the precise mechanism is unknown, excess consumption of saturated fat makes the body less sensitive to the effects of the hormone insulin, thereby contributing to insulin resistance (see page 12) and type 2 diabetes. The availability of lean meats and low-fat and fat-free dairy products makes it easy to switch from foods that are high in saturated fat to those with a lower fat content without having to give up the benefits of taste and nutrition.

Added Sugars

You may have a sweet tooth, but the added sugar in foods hurts not only your teeth but also your waistline. Sweet desserts and snacks are okay for special occasions, but on a regular basis they serve only to put on pounds while supplying few nutrients. In fact, filling up on sugary foods leaves you less hungry for foods that pack a higher nutritional punch.

Sugary soft drinks have been singled out in recent years as a possible contributor to the steep rise in the incidence of obesity and type 2 diabetes among both children and adults. The consumption of sugary soft drinks by adults rose more than 60 percent from the late 1970s to the late 1990s and more than doubled among children and adolescents. In fact, sugary soft drinks now make up about 7 percent of the total food consumption in the United States.

Soft drinks are also a major source of added sugars in our diet. Each 12-ounce can of soda contains 40 to 50 grams of sugar—about 9 teaspoons—and 160 to 200 calories. If you drink one can of soda each day and do not offset it by cutting back on your calorie intake in another way, you will gain 15 pounds in one year. Reducing your consumption of sugary, high-calorie soft drinks might be the single most effective step you can take to lose weight or to keep from becoming overweight.

Sodium

Sodium occurs naturally in many foods and is an important mineral that the body needs in small amounts to help regulate body fluids, muscle contraction, and nerve impulses. Problems arise when sodium, in the form commonly known as table salt, is added to food in excessive amounts. Food manufacturers, seeking to make their foods more flavorful and longer lasting, add most of the excess salt. But many of us also use the salt shaker to make our foods even saltier.

The cumulative effect of all this added salt can contribute to high blood pressure, which is common in people who are obese and those who have type 2 diabetes. Some people are more sensitive than others to the effects of sodium on their blood pressure, but most of us eat much more salt than the 2,300-milligram recommended daily limit. Doctors generally recommend that everyone try to cut back on their sodium intake. If you seem to be sodium-sensitive, your doctor may suggest reducing your intake to less than 1,500 milligrams of sodium a day.

Again, it's important to read food labels when you shop. You'll be surprised at how many foods contain a large amount of sodium. Buy low-sodium, reduced-sodium, or no-salt-added soups and canned vegetables. In addition to the sodium content, look for hidden salt ingredients such as monosodium glutamate and sodium nitrite. Avoid processed sandwich meats and smoked meats, which tend to be salty. For more about sodium and high blood pressure, see page 60.

Lack of Exercise

The human body was not meant to spend most hours of the day in a car, behind a desk, or in front of a television or a computer. But this has become our way of life. While technological advances provide many benefits, they can come at a high cost to our health, primarily by reducing the need for physical activity in our daily lives. The requirement for physical labor on the job is much less today than it was only a century ago, when most people engaged in physical, often back-breaking work. Walking used to be the major mode of transportation, and most household tasks, such as washing clothes and dishes, required physical exertion.

Today, about one in four American adults leads a sedentary life, which is defined as engaging in less than 30 minutes of physical activity each day. An additional one-third of adults fail to get enough exercise to achieve health benefits. By this definition, more than half of Americans are sedentary.

TV watching is probably the leading sedentary activity in the United States. Adults spend about 30 hours each week in front of the TV, and many families have several TVs in their home, complete with remote controls. Couple this lack of physical activity with the constant exposure to TV ads for unhealthy high-calorie foods and you can understand how the increase in TV watching plays a role in the rise in obesity, the major risk factor for type 2 diabetes.

In addition, a lack of physical fitness is directly related to a higher risk of death from all causes, but especially from heart disease. Physical fitness improves cardiovascular fitness, making the heart more efficient at pumping blood throughout the body. In addition, regular exercise increases the level of beneficial HDL cholesterol in the blood. HDL cholesterol carries excess cholesterol out of the arteries and back to the liver, which removes it from the body. LDL cholesterol is the harmful form of cholesterol because it can build up in the artery walls and eventually cause a heart attack or a stroke.

Smoking

Smoking cigarettes has many adverse effects on health, especially to the heart, blood vessels, and lungs. Smoking can also increase the risk of type 2 diabetes because smoking reduces the body's ability to use the hormone insulin. When cells cannot respond effectively to insulin, they do not take in glucose from the blood in sufficient amounts and the pancreas makes more and more insulin. This condition, called insulin resistance (see page 12), contributes to the development of type 2 diabetes.

In addition to reducing your body's ability to use insulin, smoking increases the level of total cholesterol and other fats in the blood, increasing your risk of heart disease, heart attack, and stroke. Smoking also restricts the amount of oxygen that reaches your cells and tissues and replaces the oxygen with harmful carbon monoxide.

Stress

The amount of daily stress you face may also put you at risk for type 2 diabetes. Some research has found that stress—and the way a person handles it—may affect levels of blood sugar and insulin (the hormone that regulates blood sugar). Stress causes the body to release so-called stress hormones, such as adrenaline and cortisol. Under normal conditions, stress hormones are helpful because they provide the needed energy to overcome a challenge or escape an immediate danger. These hormones temporarily increase the release of sugar from the liver into the bloodstream to provide energy to meet the challenge and then the liver's release of sugar drops back to normal once the challenge is met.

But when a person is under constant stress, which can result from a traumatic life event such as the death of a loved one, cortisol stays at an elevated level over time, increasing insulin resistance and the possibility of elevated blood sugar. The high level of cortisol promotes the accumulation of fat around the abdomen, and this accumulation of excess fat in the abdominal area can make the cells even less sensitive to insulin, further increasing the risk of type 2 diabetes. For many people, stress management (see page 128) can be an important way to reduce the risk of health problems.

Lack of Sleep

Some medical studies suggest that lack of sleep may also be a risk factor for type 2 diabetes. Americans have been sleeping fewer and fewer hours over the past century—from an average of 9 hours in 1900 to 6 hours or fewer today.

Sleep loss seems to affect diabetes risk in two ways: by promoting weight gain and by interfering with the way the body uses glucose. Sleep loss can cause weight gain by reducing the nightly production of growth hormone, a hormone that triggers both the manufacture of protein in muscle and the breakdown of stored fat, which in turn regulates the body's proportion of muscle to fat. A reduction in growth hormone can lead to an accumulation of fat, reduced muscle mass, and obesity, the most important risk factor for type 2 diabetes.

Lack of sleep also may interfere with the body's normal use of carbohydrates and glucose. The lack of sleep causes blood sugar levels to rise higher than usual and return to normal more slowly, and it slows the body's production of insulin. People without diabetes who sleep fewer than 4 hours a night show signs of developing impaired fasting glucose (elevated blood sugar levels) or prediabetes, the precursor to type 2 diabetes. People who routinely fail to get enough sleep also are at risk of developing insulin resistance, which contributes to type 2 diabetes.

Impaired Fasting Glucose and Impaired Glucose Tolerance

Impaired fasting glucose is a condition in which the results of a fasting blood glucose test show a blood glucose level between 100 and 125 mg/dL after a person has fasted overnight (or 12 hours). Doctors diagnose impaired glucose tolerance when a person's blood glucose levels are between 140 and 190 mg/dL 2 hours after drinking a sugary drink. These levels are above the normal glucose levels but below the level required for a diagnosis of type 2 diabetes. Impaired fasting glucose and impaired glucose tolerance are also features of insulin resistance syndrome (see page 16).

If you have been diagnosed with impaired fasting glucose or impaired glucose tolerance, you are at very high risk of developing type 2 diabetes. Your doctor will recommend measures you can take to bring your glucose level back down and reverse the progression to type 2 diabetes.

Diabetes during Pregnancy

Gestational diabetes (see chapter 15) is a form of diabetes that some women develop when they are pregnant and that usually goes away on its own after delivery. However, having diabetes during a pregnancy greatly increases a woman's probability of developing it in a future pregnancy and of developing type 2 diabetes later in life. If you have had gestational diabetes during a pregnancy, your doctor will recommend steps you can take to lower your chances of developing type 2 diabetes in the future. The children of mothers who develop diabetes during a pregnancy are also at increased risk of developing type 2 diabetes at some time in their life.

Gestational diabetes poses a more immediate threat to the fetus than to the pregnant woman. If gestational diabetes goes undiagnosed, stillbirth and newborn complications are more common than in pregnancies of women who do not develop diabetes during their pregnancy.

Polycystic Ovarian Syndrome

Polycystic ovarian syndrome is characterized by higher than normal levels of male hormones (androgens) and by the presence of many small cysts on the ovaries that do not go away on their own, as most ovarian cysts do. Most women with polycystic ovarian syndrome are overweight, although normal-weight women can also have the disorder. Whether thin or overweight, affected women tend to carry most of their weight in the abdominal area, unlike most women, who tend to carry their weight around their thighs and hips.

When cells are not responding to insulin in a normal way, the pancreas produces larger amounts of insulin to help get sugar out of the bloodstream and into the cells. In women who are at risk for polycystic ovarian syndrome, the higher levels of insulin in the blood stimulate the ovaries to produce an excessive amount of testosterone and other male hormones. The increased levels of male hormones cause the syndrome's characteristic symptoms, including the accumulation of fat around the abdomen.

Women who have polycystic ovarian syndrome typically have irregular menstrual periods and are often infertile because they don't ovulate. (Ovulation is the cyclical release of an egg from an ovary.) Polycystic ovarian syndrome is usually diagnosed when a woman seeks treatment for infertility.

Lifestyle factors—including eating a healthy diet, exercising regularly, and losing weight—can significantly reduce a woman's risk for polycystic ovarian syndrome as well as type 2 diabetes and heart disease. If you are diagnosed with polycystic ovarian syndrome, your doctor will refer you to a dietitian or a nutritionist, who can help you develop a structured diet and exercise plan that you can adapt to your daily routine.

Gum Disease

Keeping your teeth and gums healthy can pay off in many more ways than giving you a nice smile. It can also help prevent type 2 diabetes as well as heart disease and other health problems. Gum disease (see page 188), known medically as periodontal disease, is a long-recognized complication of type 2 diabetes, but many health experts now consider gum disease to also be a risk factor for type 2 diabetes.

The bacteria that cause gum disease may trigger the release of inflammatory substances by the immune system that can damage cells throughout the body, including in the pancreas, where insulin is manufactured. This process can occur even in people who have no other risk factors for type 2 diabetes.

To prevent gum disease, brush your teeth at least twice a day, floss daily, and see your dentist twice a year for a checkup and cleaning.

PART TWO

Preventing
Type 2 Diabetes

3

Maintaining a Healthy Weight

Maintaining a healthy weight is one of the most important things you can do to prevent type 2 diabetes because being overweight is a major risk factor. When you eat too much, the extra calories that are not immediately used are stored as fat. When you regularly eat too much, the stored fat that isn't used keeps accumulating.

These accumulated fat stores, especially when located in the abdominal area, somehow reduce the ability of the cells to respond to the hormone insulin, interrupting the normal process of energy use by the cells. This condition in which the cells are less sensitive to insulin is called insulin resistance (see page 12). Insulin normally enables cells to take in glucose from the blood to use or store for future use. The pancreas responds to insulin resistance by making more insulin. If the pancreas cannot make enough insulin to overcome the cells' resistance, blood sugar rises. If blood sugar continues to rise, type 2 diabetes eventually develops.

If you are at risk for type 2 diabetes, losing weight is probably the most important step you can take to avoid it. If you have insulin resistance, losing weight can reverse it by making your cells more sensitive to insulin. Even if you are not overweight, you should eat a healthy diet and get regular exercise to help prevent the weight gain that often accompanies aging.

Are You Overweight?

Two factors determine whether you weigh too much: the number of pounds you weigh and the percentage of your body that is made up of fat. The distribution of fat on your body is also important. People who carry more weight in the abdominal area than on their hips and thighs have a higher risk of developing not only type 2 diabetes but also high blood pressure, heart disease, and stroke.

To check your weight status, use the body mass index (BMI) chart below. Body mass index is calculated with a mathematical formula in which your body weight in kilograms is divided by the square of your height in meters. The BMI is an excellent, although not perfect, indicator of the percentage of body fat. A BMI of 18.5 to 24.9 is considered healthy. A BMI of 25 to 29.9 signals overweight and an increased risk of health problems. People who have a BMI of 30 or more are considered obese. Most people who have type 2 diabetes are overweight or obese.

In general, a woman whose waist size is larger than 35 inches and a man whose waist is larger than 40 inches are at increased risk for type 2 diabetes because waist size signals the accumulation of fat within the abdomen. Fat stored in the abdomen has a greater influence on insulin sensitivity than fat stored elsewhere on the body.

Body mass index (BMI) is a method of evaluating your health status based on your weight. When you are overweight, you store more fat on your body in relation to muscle; the added fat puts you at risk for health conditions such as type 2 diabetes and heart disease. The BMI uses your height and weight to evaluate body fat, which doctors consider a helpful indicator of health risks. Athletes and bodybuilders are exceptions to this general rule; they often have a high BMI but, because they have more muscle than fat on their body, they have fewer health risks. However, for most people, the higher the BMI, the higher the health risks.

Q&A

Q. What is a calorie?

A. A calorie is a unit of energy contained in food. The number of calories you need each day to maintain your current weight varies according to your gender, size, and activity level. In general, inactive women need to consume about 1,600 calories a day. Physically active women require around 2,200 daily calories, about the same number as inactive men. Active men need to take in roughly 2,800 calories per day. The calorie requirements of active men and women are even higher if they are training for competitions such as marathons or triathlons.

If you want to lose weight, remember that to lose 1 pound in a week you need to eat 500 fewer calories each day, or 3,500 fewer calories each week. Or you need to burn 500 more calories each day. A good calorie-reducing approach is to plan more meals around vegetables, whole grains, legumes, and fruits.

Finding Your BMI

To determine your BMI, find your height in the left column and read across the row to find your weight. Scan to the bottom of your weight column to find your BMI. A healthy BMI ranges from 18.5 to 24.9. A person whose BMI is 25 to 29.9 is considered overweight. A BMI of 30 or higher indicates obesity.

BODY MASS INDEX (KILOGRAMS PER SQUARE METER)

Height	Body Weight (pounds)													
4'10"	91	96	100	105	110	115	119	124	129	134	138	143	167	191
4'11"	94	99	104	109	114	119	124	128	133	138	143	148	173	198
5'	97	102	107	112	118	123	128	133	138	143	148	153	179	204
5'1"	100	106	111	116	122	127	132	137	143	148	153	158	185	211
5'2"	104	109	115	120	126	131	136	142	147	153	158	164	191	218
5'3"	107	113	118	124	130	135	141	146	152	158	163	169	197	225
5'4"	110	116	122	128	134	140	145	151	157	163	169	174	204	232
5'5"	114	120	126	132	138	144	150	156	162	168	174	180	210	240
5'6"	118	124	130	136	142	148	155	161	167	173	179	186	216	247
5'7"	121	127	134	140	146	153	159	166	172	178	185	191	223	255
5'8"	125	131	138	144	151	158	164	171	177	184	190	197	230	262
5'9"	128	135	142	149	155	162	169	176	182	189	196	203	236	270
5'10"	132	139	146	153	160	167	174	181	188	195	202	209	243	278
5'11"	136	143	150	157	165	172	179	186	193	200	208	215	250	286
6'	140	147	154	162	169	177	184	191	199	206	213	221	258	294
6'1"	144	151	159	166	174	182	189	197	204	212	219	227	265	302
6'2"	148	155	163	171	179	186	194	202	210	218	225	233	272	311
6'3"	152	160	168	176	184	192	200	208	216	224	232	240	279	319
6'4"	156	164	172	180	189	197	205	213	221	230	238	246	287	328
BMI	19	20	21	22	23	24	25	26	27	28	29	30	35	40

Key: Underweight (less than 18.5)   Healthy weight (18.5 to 24.9)   Overweight (25 to 29.9)   Obese (30 and above)

Losing Weight Sensibly

There are a variety of ways to lose weight, but the difficult part is keeping the weight off once you lose it. The best way to lose weight successfully is to adopt healthy eating and exercise habits you can maintain for the rest of your life. This may not be as hard as you think. For example, giving up your daily can of pop—which contains 9 teaspoons of sugar—can save 150 calories each day. Those calories add up to 54,750 calories for the year. Making just this one change may enable you to lose as many as 15 pounds in a year, provided that you don't substitute your soft drink for something else with a similar number of calories.

Health experts have found that even a small weight loss—5 to 7 percent of your body weight (that's 10 to 14 pounds if you weigh 200 pounds)—delivers health benefits, especially if you are at risk for type 2 diabetes. Weight loss can make your cells more sensitive to the effects of insulin, thereby helping to reduce blood sugar.

Sensible weight loss means losing ½ to 1 pound per week—you're more likely to keep it off over the long term. To lose 1 pound in a week, you need to eat 3,500 fewer calories than you burn in a week. That's 500 calories each day.

Diets that completely eliminate certain food groups are popular but can be harmful because they do not provide all of the nutrients your body needs. For example, diets that exclude carbohydrates don't provide the vitamins, minerals, and antioxidants contained in fruits, vegetables, and whole grains. They also fail to supply sufficient fiber, a nutrient that helps keep the blood sugar level steady.

Although high-protein diets can result in rapid weight loss, at least initially, they can raise blood cholesterol levels because they are often high in saturated fat. Like all diets that eliminate certain food groups, the weight loss from high-protein diets comes more from cutting calories than from eating mostly protein. In addition, the initial weight loss usually comes from the loss of water. Restrictive diets tend to work better in the short run and rarely produce sustainable weight loss over time.

Doctors know that the only dependable way to lose weight is to eat less and exercise more. That means that you will have to cut your intake of calories while increasing your physical activity. You're more likely to keep your weight off over the long term if you lose about 1 pound a week.

Make an Eating Plan

Very restrictive diets are often hard to maintain, and people tend to start gaining back the weight as soon as the diet ends. It's much more sensible to follow a reasonable diet plan that you can stick to for the rest of your life.

A diabetes-fighting diet is heart-healthy, calorie-conscious, high in fiber and other important nutrients, and low in harmful fats and sweets. Specifically, it is rich in whole grains, vegetables, legumes, and fruits, and replaces unhealthy fats (such as those in fatty meats and snack foods) with healthy plant-based fats (such as olive oil) and omega-3 fatty acids (from fish).

Work with your doctor or a dietitian to come up with an eating plan that will help you lose weight. A healthy, effective weight-loss diet will have the following important components:

The Right Number of Calories Strive to cut your calorie intake by 20 percent. Your daily calorie allowance is 12 to 15 times your current weight, depending on whether you are inactive or active. For example, if you weigh 180 pounds and you are inactive, your daily calorie count is 180×12, or 2,160 calories; if you are active, your daily calorie count is 180×15, or 2,700. To cut those calories by 20 percent, multiply them by 0.8: $2,160 \times 0.8 = 1,728$ calories; $2,700 \times 0.8 = 2,160$. That is your daily calorie allowance for losing weight. As you lose weight, you will need to adjust your calorie intake downward so you continue to lose weight. Check food labels and recipes for calorie counts per serving.

Enough Vitamins and Minerals To make sure you're getting enough of these important nutrients, the biggest share of your daily calories should come from vegetables, fruits, and whole grains. (And just to be safe, you might consider taking a multivitamin/mineral supplement every day.)

Adequate Protein Women need less than 50 grams of protein daily and men require less than 60 grams. Good protein sources

Don't Skip Breakfast

Evidence shows that people who eat breakfast are nearly half as likely to become obese and develop diabetes as those who don't eat breakfast regularly. Although doctors are not sure exactly why this is, they think it may be because breakfast jump-starts your metabolism, helping you burn more calories throughout the day. Also, because breakfast curbs hunger, it may help keep you from overeating later in the day.

But make sure your morning meal is nutritious. Skip the doughnuts and coffee cake. Instead, have a fiber-rich cereal with skim milk and a piece of fruit or a hard-boiled egg and a slice of whole-grain toast (dry or with a plant sterol spread, not butter or stick margarine made with trans fats). If you're pressed for time, have some leftovers from last night's dinner. Anything nutritious is better than no breakfast at all.

include lean meats, poultry without the skin, fish, legumes (dried beans and peas), and fat-free dairy products.

Enough Carbohydrates   You need to consume about 55 percent of your total calorie intake from carbohydrate-rich foods. If you are on a 1,600-calorie diet, this means taking in just over 200 grams of carbohydrates. Again, make sure they come in the form of whole grains (breads, rice, pasta, and cereals), vegetables, and fruits.

Limited Fat   Keep your intake of dietary fat below 30 percent of total calories per day and make sure that most of those fats are monounsaturated and polyunsaturated (see page 49). Limit saturated fats (found in meats, butter, and full-fat dairy products) to less than 10 percent of total daily calories and try to avoid trans fats (found in stick margarine, baked goods, and other foods that contain partially hydrogenated vegetable oils).

Losing Weight by Limiting Fat

If you are thinking about limiting any food group for quicker weight loss, consider reducing or eliminating saturated and trans fats. You'll be cutting the unhealthy, artery-clogging fats and probably be cutting calories at the same time. But keep in mind that to lose weight, you must not increase your intake of other kinds of foods to replace the fatty foods you are limiting. Fat has more than twice as many calories per gram as carbohydrates and protein do—9 calories per gram for fat versus 4 calories per gram for carbs and protein. Here's how to reduce your intake of saturated and trans fats:

- Don't consume full-fat dairy products such as butter, ice cream, and whole milk.
- Trim all visible fat from meat and remove the skin from poultry before serving.
- Don't use stick margarine. Choose tub margarines that contain plant sterols or stanols, naturally occurring substances in plants that can significantly reduce cholesterol levels when consumed regularly.
- Use liquid vegetable oils (such as olive and canola) for cooking and salad dressings. Plant-based unsaturated fats can actually improve cholesterol levels.

Watch Portion Sizes

Over the past decade, Americans have been eating more and more of their meals in restaurants, ordering takeout and delivery for family dinners, and picking up fast-food meals on their way home from work. As a result, it is increasingly difficult to control the quantity and quality of the food we eat. The portion sizes of restaurant meals and fast foods, soft drinks, and baked goods such as muffins, cookies, and bagels have grown huge. As portion sizes get bigger, so do our waistlines and our risk of developing type 2 diabetes, high blood pressure, heart disease, cancer, and other health problems.

There is a difference between a portion and a serving. A portion is the amount of food you choose to eat, large or small. A serving is a measured amount of a food or a dish, which can be standardized by the government, as on a food label, or established in a recipe, a cookbook, or by your dietitian's meal plan. The portion of rice that you are used to eating, for example, may be two or three times the standard serving size indicated on the rice package.

Learning to recognize standard serving sizes can help you judge how much you are eating and help you limit your portions and calories if you are trying to lose weight. Here are some tips for helping you control portion size:

- Check the number of servings in the package listed on the Nutrition Facts panel of the food label. For example, if there are four servings in a package and one serving provides 100 calories and you eat the whole package, you are consuming four servings and 400 calories, not 100 calories.

- Compare your usual portion sizes to those on food labels.

- Pay attention to what you are eating. Enjoy the taste, smell, and texture of the food you are eating to make the experience last longer.

- Eat slowly so your brain has time to receive the message that you are getting full.

- Put more vegetables, legumes, and whole grains on your plate than meat, and have fruit for dessert.

- Don't skip meals, especially breakfast. You may end up eating more high-calorie foods at the next meal.

- At a restaurant, share your meal with a friend or take half of it home for another meal.

- Avoid "value" and supersize meals at fast-food restaurants.

- Use your hand to eyeball portion sizes:

  Palm = 3 ounces of meat, poultry, or fish

  Fist = 1 medium fruit or 1 cup of cut-up fruit

  Cupped hand = 1 to 2 ounces of nuts

  Thumb (base to tip) = 1 ounce of meat or cheese

- Read food labels. Watch for trans fats and partially hydrogenated oils in snack chips, crackers, and cookies as well as in some more surprising places such as chicken broth, low-fat ice cream, microwave popcorn, and bread.

- Don't cook or bake with vegetable shortening, which is a hydrogenated oil.

Counting Fat Grams

Counting fat grams is an alternative to counting calories when you're trying to lose weight. When you limit the amount of fat in your diet, you are also likely to reduce the number of calories you consume. Here are some guidelines to help you lose weight by limiting the amount of fat—counted in grams—in your diet:

- First, calculate the number of calories you need to consume to maintain your current weight. You do this by multiplying your weight in pounds by 12 if you are not active or 15 if you are active. Let's say you weigh 180 pounds. If you are inactive, you consume about 2,160 (180 × 12 = 2,160) calories a day to maintain your weight. If you are active, you consume about 2,700 (180 × 15 = 2,700) calories each day to maintain your weight.

- To lose weight, you need to eat 250 to 1,000 fewer calories each day. If you reduce your daily calorie consumption by 500 calories, for example, your daily calorie count would be 1,660 to 2,200 calories, depending on your level of activity. Remember that increasing your level of activity as you eat fewer calories can significantly boost your weight-loss efforts.

- The chart below shows the daily limit of total fat grams and saturated fat grams based on daily calorie intake. You should limit your total fat intake to less than 30 percent of calories and your saturated fat intake to 7 to 10 percent of total calories. Find your daily calorie intake in the left column and look across the row to find your total daily fat gram limit and the 10- and 7-percent limits of saturated fat grams. If your calorie intake is, say, 1,800, you should eat fewer than 60 grams of total fat, and of that 60 grams, fewer than 20 grams should be from saturated fat (if you're limiting it to 10 percent) or 14 grams (for a 7-percent saturated fat limit).

- Read food labels to find out how many fat grams and calories are in the foods you eat. A good rule of thumb for identifying low-fat foods is to look for 3 or fewer grams of fat for every 100 calories in a serving.

- Remember to eat mostly healthy fats: polyunsaturated and monounsaturated fats and plant sterols (in some tub margarines and salad dressings).

DAILY FAT GRAM LIMITS (AS PERCENTAGE OF DAILY CALORIES)

Total Calories	Total Fat Grams 30% or Less	Saturated Fat Grams 10% or Less	Saturated Fat Grams 7% or Less
1,200	40 or fewer	13 or fewer	9 or fewer
1,500	50 or fewer	17 or fewer	12 or fewer
1,800	60 or fewer	20 or fewer	14 or fewer
2,000	67 or fewer	22 or fewer	16 or fewer
2,200	73 or fewer	24 or fewer	17 or fewer
2,500	83 or fewer	28 or fewer	19 or fewer
3,000	100 or fewer	33 or fewer	23 or fewer

Developing Healthy Eating Habits

One good way to ensure that the weight you lose stays off is to adopt healthy eating habits that you can follow for the rest of your life. This probably means changing the way you buy and consume food—in fact, it may even mean changing your whole relationship with eating and food. We live in a culture that encourages us to consume more food than our body needs. Many of us have an emotional attachment to food—eating our favorite "comfort foods," for example, makes us feel good. Some of us eat when we're sad or bored, often without realizing why we're doing it. In these situations, we are often making unhealthy food choices and taking in too many calories.

You need to be able to control the food environment you live in. Recognizing the situations that make you want to eat is an important step toward taking control of and changing your eating habits. Here are some helpful guidelines for improving your eating habits and your relationship with food:

- Eat only when you're hungry.
- Eat slowly. It takes 20 to 30 minutes to start feeling full.
- Stop eating *before* you are full.
- Begin meals with a large glass of water.
- Fill half of your plate with vegetables. Devote one-quarter to a protein source and one-quarter to a starchy food such as brown rice or another whole grain.
- Keep a food diary. Note the type and amount of food you eat and how you felt before you began eating. This information will help you keep track of what and how much you're eating, understand your eating habits, and provide clues to your emotional relationship with food.
- Eat in only one room of your house. Eating in the same room cuts down on snacking and grazing.
- Eat only at certain times of the day. A good approach is to eat three small meals and two snacks every day rather than three large meals.
- Identify your eating triggers—the times or situations that make you most likely to lose control over your eating. If it is at night after the kids go to bed and you watch TV, try to change your

routine by, for example, reading a book instead of watching TV. If the worst time is after work, going for a walk or to the gym can help you break the after-work eat-everything-in-sight habit when you get home.

- Don't buy tempting cookies, candy, and snack foods. If they're not in the house, you won't have to force yourself to resist them.
- Never shop when you're hungry. You're more likely to buy your favorite high-calorie snacks.

Commercial Weight-Loss Programs

If you have tried to lose weight on your own without success, a commercial weight-loss program may help you lose weight more easily and keep it off. Such programs often provide structure, education, and support. Some may even be claimed as a medical deduction on income tax returns. Just make sure that the program is reputable, has a proven success rate, and is tailored to your needs—and always talk to your doctor before starting on a commercial weight-loss plan. Keep in mind that to maintain any weight loss over the long term, you have to incorporate lifestyle changes, such as increasing your level of physical activity, that you can follow throughout your life.

Weight-loss plans offer a variety of approaches to dieting, including prepackaged meals, portion-control advice, weight-loss medication, or liquid meals. Their strategies may include goal-setting, meal plans, shopping lists, accountability tracking, food journals, and weight-loss tips. Study a plan's materials carefully to determine whether a given approach might work for you. Many plans have a Web site that provides preliminary information to help people decide if their approach seems like the best fit for them. If you have any questions about a given plan, talk to your doctor or a registered dietitian.

Healthy Weight-Loss Strategies

Work actively with your doctor to come up with strategies to help you change the way you eat, not just the amount. The following approaches can help you cut back on your calorie intake:

- **Eat more fiber.** Make an effort to eat more fruits, vegetables, whole grains, and legumes. Fiber helps slow down the rate at which glucose enters the blood.

- **Don't skip meals.** Skipping a meal can make you overeat later in the day. Instead, eat three small meals a day and two snacks at regular intervals.

- **Make healthy substitutions.** Eat a piece of fruit instead of potato chips for a snack. Buy fat-free sour cream and low-fat cheeses. Drink water instead of sugary soft drinks or alcohol.

- **Eat smaller portions.** Keep your meal portions sensible. Enjoy a small amount of a favorite indulgence food every so often so you don't feel deprived or get discouraged while you're dieting.

- **Avoid eating triggers.** If the bakery or the fast-food restaurant on the way home tempts you, take a different route.

Tips for Eating Out

Eating out can be challenging when you're trying to lose weight. You may be dining with friends or family who encourage you to go off your diet "just this once." To keep on track, use these tips for healthy—and sensible—eating out:

- Skip the cocktail. Alcohol contains a lot of calories and few nutrients. Instead, order sparkling water with a slice of lemon or lime, iced tea, or fat-free milk.

- Don't be reluctant to ask the waiter questions about ingredients and how a dish is prepared or request a special preparation, such as grilled instead of fried.

- Don't fill up on bread or crackers while waiting for your meal.

- Order a low-fat, low-calorie appetizer and a salad instead of an entrée for a meal.

- Split a meal with a friend or a family member or take half home for later.

- Order meat, fish, or poultry that is steamed, broiled, poached, roasted, or baked without fat. Choose or request skinless cuts of poultry. Squeeze lemon on top for added flavor.

- Avoid dishes whose descriptions include words or terms that indicate higher fat, such as fried, buttered, creamed, gravy, cheese sauce, au gratin, scalloped, rich, pastry, or cooked in oil.

- Avoid dishes whose descriptions include words or terms that indicate higher salt, such as smoked, pickled, broth, barbecued, cocktail sauce, tomato sauce, mustard sauce, soy sauce, teriyaki, or marinated.

- Have a large salad as a main course, with low-fat dressing or olive oil and vinegar on the side. Avoid the high-calorie, high-fat add-ons, such as cheese and bacon.
- Tell the server to hold the gravy, sauce, butter, and other fat-laden toppings.
- If you go to a fast-food restaurant, skip the fried foods and order a grilled chicken sandwich (no mayo) with a side salad and water or low-fat milk.
- Have fresh fruit for dessert.

4

Nutrition Basics for Staying Healthy

Consuming a healthy and balanced diet is one of the most important things you can do to avoid type 2 diabetes. Because being overweight is a major risk factor for type 2 diabetes, a diabetes-fighting diet is moderate in calories. And because heart disease and high blood pressure risks often coincide with type 2 diabetes risk, a diabetes-prevention diet should be low in fat, especially artery-clogging saturated fats and trans fats, and sodium. The bottom line for achieving these goals: eat more fresh foods, especially vegetables, fruits, and whole grains, and less red meat, cheese, rich desserts, and processed foods. The information in this chapter can help you adopt a healthy eating plan that you can follow for the rest of your life.

What Is a Healthy Diet?

To eat healthfully, choose a wide variety of nutritious foods every day—and don't be reluctant to try new foods. Variety is the best way to get all the nutrients your body needs. But you need to watch out for foods that are calorie-dense and choose foods that are nutrient-dense—those that pack lots of nutrients relative to their calorie count. Limit high-calorie, nutrient-poor foods such as fast foods, bakery goods, candy, sugary soft drinks, and snack foods such as chips.

If your doctor has told you that you are at risk of developing type 2 diabetes, he or she will work with you to develop a diet plan that fits your lifestyle and daily routine. Here are some of the most important dietary recommendations that you can follow:

- Consume from 5 to 13 servings of fruits and vegetables every day. Studies have shown that people who eat 10 servings of fruits and vegetables a day can significantly reduce their risk of having a stroke.

- Limit saturated fats (found in red meats, poultry skin, and full-fat dairy products) and avoid trans fats altogether (check package labels). Specifically, limit your total daily fat intake to less than 30 percent of your total daily calories, limit saturated fat to less than 10 percent of your total daily calories, and limit dietary cholesterol to 300 milligrams each day (200 milligrams if you have heart disease).

- Limit your intake of sugary foods (including sugary soft drinks, cakes, pies, doughnuts, cookies, and candy) because they contain lots of calories but few nutrients.

- Boost your intake of fiber. The best sources are vegetables, fruits, whole grains, and legumes (dried beans, peas, and lentils).

- Limit your intake of sodium to 2,300 milligrams each day.

- Use low-fat cooking methods such as baking, broiling, grilling, steaming, or poaching. Use cooking sprays for stir-fries and sautéing.

- Balance the calories you take in with those you burn through exercise.

Getting the Important Nutrients

Most foods are made up of three basic components: carbohydrates, fat, and protein. Carbohydrates—composed of simple and complex sugars—are the body's most important source of fuel. Because of their importance, carbohydrates should comprise 50 to 65 percent of your daily intake of calories. Fats (primarily from vegetable fats) should comprise no more than 30 percent of your daily calories, and protein should supply the rest, usually 12 to 20 percent.

Carbohydrates

Plant foods provide the sugars, starches, and fiber that make up the carbohydrate category of foods. Carbohydrates are classified as simple or complex. Examples of simple carbohydrates include table sugar (sucrose), the sugar found in fruit (fructose), and the milk sugar lactose. Simple carbohydrates are generally sweet-tasting and easily digestible. Because they are digested rapidly, they can cause a rapid rise in blood sugar levels.

Foods containing simple carbohydrates or starches that are quickly broken down into sugar—such as white bread and white rice—tend to be highly refined. When a grain is refined, the fiber-rich outer bran and the nutritious inner germ of the grain are removed, leaving mostly the starchy inside of the seed. This starchy substance is digested fast and sent to the bloodstream, causing blood sugar to spike. For this reason, if you have elevated blood sugar levels, you need to minimize your intake of simple sugars or consume other foods such as protein at the same time to counteract their effect on your blood sugar.

Complex carbohydrates—found in whole-grain foods such as brown rice and whole-wheat bread and pasta, vegetables, fruits with their skin, and legumes (dried peas, beans, and lentils)—should make up the bulk of your carbohydrate intake. Your bloodstream absorbs the nutrients from complex carbohydrates more slowly than it does those from simple carbohydrates. Foods containing complex carbohydrates also supply more vitamins and minerals than those containing simple carbohydrates.

Fiber

Fiber, a substance found in the cell walls of plants, is a type of carbohydrate that is especially important in the diets of people who are at risk of developing type 2 diabetes. A diet high in fiber-rich foods can help make the cells more sensitive to insulin, which regulates blood sugar levels. Eating high-fiber foods has other benefits, too, such as helping lower artery-clogging LDL cholesterol in the blood, thereby reducing the risk of heart disease.

A good rule of thumb for lowering heart disease risk is to eat 14 grams of fiber for every 1,000 calories you consume. For a 2,000-calorie-a-day diet, that translates into 28 grams of fiber each day. This may be more than you are used to and therefore will require significant changes in your eating habits. If you haven't been consuming many high-fiber foods, increase your intake gradually to prevent intestinal gas and bloating. Drink at least 8 glasses of water daily because eating a lot of fiber without taking in enough fluids can cause constipation. See the tips below for how to include more fiber in your diet.

There are two types of fiber—water-soluble and water-insoluble—both of which serve vital functions in the body. Soluble fiber slows down the rate at which the small intestine releases glucose into the bloodstream, leveling out the highs and lows in blood glucose concentration, and also improves blood cholesterol levels. Good sources of soluble fiber include oats and oat bran; barley; dried beans and peas (legumes); fruits such as apples, pears, bananas, and oranges; vegetables such as carrots, cabbage, and sweet potatoes; flaxseed; and psyllium husk (a grass found in some stool softeners and fiber supplements).

Insoluble fiber softens and gives bulk to stool, helping it pass more easily through the intestines. Its positive effects on bowel regularity may also help reduce the risk of colon cancer and other digestive disorders. Good sources of insoluble fiber include root vegetables; whole grains; the edible skin of fruits; vegetables such as green beans, cauliflower, and potato skins; and flaxseed.

An additional benefit of fiber is that it makes you feel full so you won't be as hungry for high-calorie snacks or sweets. Here are some tips for boosting the fiber in your diet:

- Consume whole fruits instead of fruit juices. Have fruit for snacks and dessert.
- Eat more raw vegetables, such as carrots, celery, and cucumbers, and cooked vegetables, such as broccoli and winter squash, at lunch and dinner.
- Substitute whole-grain breads and cereals, whole-wheat pasta, and brown rice for white breads, refined cereals, white pasta, and white rice.
- Make several meals meatless every week by, for example, replacing meat-based main dishes with bean-based entrées.
- Add beans, peas, and lentils to soups and salads.
- Eat oatmeal (but not the instant kind, which provides little or no fiber or other nutrients) for breakfast instead of eggs.
- Eat high-fiber cold breakfast cereals. Check the label on the cereal box for fiber content and buy only those that have 5 grams of fiber or more per serving and list whole wheat, oats, bran, barley, or any other whole grain first on the ingredient list.

Eat Your Fruits and Veggies

We have all heard from experts that eating at least 5 servings of fruits and vegetables each day is one of the most important things we can do for our health, but only one out of four of us is actually following this modest recommendation. And now we're being told to eat up to 13 servings of fruits and vegetables a day for good health.

Fruits and vegetables provide a wide assortment of vitamins and minerals, including the antioxidant vitamins—vitamin C, the carotenoids (beta carotene, lycopene, and lutein), and vitamin E—which fight free radicals, cell-damaging molecules that play a role in aging and most chronic diseases, including type 2 diabetes.

Fruits and vegetables also provide fiber, an essential nutrient that promotes healthy bowel function and helps lower the risk of heart disease and some types of cancer. They are so good-tasting and so good for you that you should try to consume as many as you can. Five

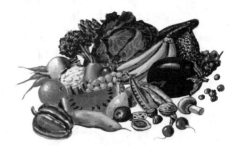

servings a day is the minimum—13 a day is better—for keeping you healthy. Here are some tips to help you get your daily dose of fruits and veggies:

- Have one or two servings of fruit at breakfast.
- Choose a fruit or a vegetable for a snack.
- Have a salad at lunch.
- Stock up on dried, canned, and frozen fruits (no sugar added) and vegetables.
- Serve more than one vegetable at dinner.

Fat

Fats add flavor and smoothness to the food you eat. They also make you feel fuller and make cakes and other baked goods soft. There are several types of naturally occurring fats in food: monounsaturated fats, polyunsaturated fats (including omega-3 and omega-6 fatty acids), saturated fats, cholesterol, and plant sterols.

The chart on page 52 highlights the differences between these dietary fats, their major food sources, and how they affect cholesterol levels in the blood.

Healthy Fats

In the past, all fats were condemned as generally unhealthy, but now we know that, in moderation, some fats are good for us. These beneficial fats help the body store energy, absorb and transport the fat-soluble vitamins (such as A, D, E, and K), and manufacture some hormones. The healthiest fats are monounsaturated and polyunsaturated fats and plant sterols.

Monounsaturated Fats

Monounsaturated fats, found mostly in olive, canola, and peanut oils, are the healthiest fats you can eat. They lower the level of total cholesterol in the blood, decrease harmful LDL cholesterol in the blood, and raise beneficial HDL cholesterol in the blood. Monounsaturated fats are usually liquid at room temperature.

Polyunsaturated Fats

Polyunsaturated fats are found in corn, sunflower, safflower, flaxseed, and soybean oils, and in the oils of fatty fish such as salmon, mackerel, and tuna. Rich in omega-3 fatty acids and omega-6 fatty acids, polyunsaturated fats lower total cholesterol in the blood, but in large amounts they can also lower heart-healthy HDL cholesterol. Like monounsaturated fats, polyunsaturated fats are usually liquid at room temperature.

Plant Sterols

Substances called plant sterols are a type of fat found in nuts, seeds, and many other plant foods. When eaten regularly, plant sterols can slow the absorption of dietary cholesterol and substantially lower the level of total cholesterol and harmful LDL cholesterol in the blood. Plant sterols are added to many tub margarines and salad dressings—check labels.

Harmful Fats

Saturated and trans fats are the ones you have to watch out for. These fats raise the risk of heart disease, blood vessel problems, and stroke. Dietary cholesterol, although not quite as harmful as saturated fats and trans fats, can also affect cholesterol levels. These fats are in many foods so you need to make an extra effort to limit or avoid them.

Saturated Fats

Saturated fats are found in meat, dark meat poultry and poultry skin, butter, full-fat dairy products, coconut oil, and palm oil. Saturated fats make the cells less sensitive to insulin, the hormone that regulates blood sugar. When the cells are resistant to insulin, blood glucose levels can eventually rise, increasing the risk of type 2 diabetes. Saturated fats also raise the level of total cholesterol and harmful LDL cholesterol in the blood, increasing the risk of high blood pressure and heart disease. Limit these fats to less than 10 percent of your total daily calories.

Trans Fats

Trans fats seem to be even more harmful than saturated fats. Trans fats are vegetable oils that have undergone a process called hydrogenation, which increases the shelf life and maintains the flavor of the foods to which they are added. Trans fats increase total blood cholesterol and harmful LDL cholesterol even more than saturated fats do. Trans fats

Fat Checking: Beware of Trans Fats

Scientific research has implicated trans fats, also known as trans fatty acids and hydrogenated oils, in the development of type 2 diabetes and heart disease. Trans fats are a man-made fat created when food manufacturers add hydrogen to vegetable oil, a process called hydrogenation. The vegetable oils subjected to this process are called hydrogenated or partially hydrogenated oils. In the process, the liquid oils are usually turned into solid or semisolid fats.

Manufacturers developed the hydrogenation process because it lengthened the shelf life and maintained the flavor of many foods. Partially hydrogenated oils, such as vegetable shortening, are found in a wide variety of food products in grocery stores, including snack crackers and chips; doughnuts, cookies, and many other baked goods; and some breakfast cereals. Margarine, especially in stick form, is a major source of trans fats. Restaurant fast foods deep-fried in partially hydrogenated oils—including french fries, breaded chicken, and fish—also contain large amounts of trans fats.

When it became known that saturated fat was bad for the heart, many food manufacturers substituted hydrogenated oils for butter in their products, but the hydrogenated oils have proved to be worse. Trans fats are twice as harmful to your heart as saturated fat. The mechanism by which trans fats increase diabetes risk works two ways. First, trans fats worsen the ratio of harmful LDL cholesterol to helpful HDL cholesterol—they increase the level of bad LDL cholesterol and lower the level of

good HDL cholesterol. This effect on LDL and HDL is double that of the effect of saturated fats on these two forms of cholesterol in the blood. Second, trans fats boost the level of potentially harmful fats called triglycerides in the blood. Triglycerides have been linked to an increased risk of both heart disease and diabetes.

As of January 1, 2006, food manufacturers were required to list trans fats on food nutrition labels (see page 66) along with other fats. Read food labels carefully and consistently when you're shopping and make an effort to resist foods containing trans fats. Here are some tips for avoiding trans fats:

- Read all food labels in the grocery store, especially on packaged foods such as bakery items and snack foods. Look for the words "trans fats" under the "Fat" heading, and the words "hydrogenated" or "partially hydrogenated" on the ingredients list, and don't buy items that contain these harmful fats.

- Ask before you order. When eating out, ask the waiter if the oils used in food preparation are hydrogenated or partially hydrogenated. Nonhydrogenated is best.

- Avoid stick margarines with hydrogenated fats. Buy only margarines whose labels say they contain no trans fats or hydrogenated fats. Better yet, look for tub margarines with added plant sterols, which actually improve cholesterol levels.

- Don't use hardened vegetable shortenings in cooking or baking.

are common in stick margarines; shortenings; many baked goods and packaged, processed, and fast foods; and fried foods such as french fries. Because trans fats are so harmful, doctors recommend that people try to avoid them altogether. Check the labels of packaged foods for the trans fat content and look for the terms "hydrogenated" or "partially hydrogenated" in ingredient lists, which indicate the presence of trans fats.

Dietary Cholesterol

Dietary cholesterol is present only in foods of animal origin, including egg yolks, liver and other organ meats, shellfish, full-fat dairy products, and meat and poultry. Dietary cholesterol can increase cholesterol in the blood but not as significantly as saturated fats and trans fats do. You should limit your daily intake of cholesterol to less than 300 milligrams a day, or 200 milligrams if you have heart disease.

How Dietary Fats Affect Blood Cholesterol

The cholesterol in your body is a substance made by the liver that helps the body produce hormones and bile (a fluid that aids the digestive

DIETARY FATS AND BLOOD CHOLESTEROL

Type of Fat	Main Food Sources	Effects on Blood Cholesterol
Monounsaturated fats	Most nuts, olive oil, canola oil, peanut oil, avocados	Lowers total and bad LDL cholesterol; raises good HDL cholesterol
Polyunsaturated fats	Sunflower oil, corn oil, safflower oil, flaxseed oil, soybean oil, cottonseed oil, fish	Lowers total cholesterol, but in large amounts can also lower good HDL cholesterol
Omega-3 fatty acids	Oily, coldwater fish, including salmon, tuna, lake trout, mackerel, and herring; flaxseed; wheat germ; canola oil	Lowers total cholesterol and bad LDL cholesterol
Plant sterols and stanols	Added to some tub margarines and salad dressings; occurs naturally in fruits, vegetables, nuts, cereals, and soybean oil	Lowers total cholesterol and bad LDL cholesterol
Saturated fats	Fatty red meat, dark meat and skin of poultry, full-fat and 2% (reduced-fat) dairy products, butter, coconut oil, palm oil	Raises total cholesterol and bad LDL cholesterol
Trans fats	Stick margarines, vegetable shortening, partially hydrogenated vegetable oils, some prepared and packaged baked goods and snacks including chips and crackers, some fast foods, some breakfast cereals	Raises total cholesterol and bad LDL cholesterol; may lower good HDL cholesterol
Dietary cholesterol	Egg yolks, shrimp and other shellfish, liver and other organ meats, full-fat dairy products	Raises total cholesterol, but not as much as saturated fats and trans fats do

process). Your liver manufactures most of your cholesterol, but some is absorbed into the bloodstream from the foods you eat that contain fat, particularly saturated fat and trans fats. For this reason, doctors recommend limiting your intake of these fats.

Q&A

Q. What's the difference between the cholesterol I eat and the cholesterol in my blood?

A. Dietary cholesterol refers to the cholesterol that is present is some foods—but only foods of animal origin, not plant-based foods. Common food sources of cholesterol include egg yolks, shrimp, lobster, red meat, and full-fat dairy products. The cholesterol you eat doesn't necessarily become cholesterol in your blood. Your liver produces the cholesterol that circulates in your blood. This type of cholesterol is essential for many functions in the body, including making some hormones. But if you eat too much saturated fat and trans fats, LDL (the harmful type of cholesterol) can build up inside your artery walls. This buildup of fatty deposits can eventually lead to heart disease, heart attack, and stroke. When you go to the doctor for a cholesterol test (see page 94), your doctor measures the total amount of cholesterol and the various forms of cholesterol—HDL (the good cholesterol), LDL, and triglycerides—circulating in your bloodstream. Total cholesterol readings between 120 and 199 milligrams per deciliter (mg/dL) are considered healthy.

Q. On my last cholesterol test report, I noticed a new term: triglycerides. What are triglycerides?

A. Triglycerides are a chemical form of fat that is found both in foods and in the body. The triglycerides in your blood come from two sources: from the fats you consume in food and from the triglycerides your liver makes from fats that circulate in your bloodstream.

Your body changes the extra calories you consume, those that are not used up right away, into triglycerides and the bloodstream transports them to fat cells for storage. As your body requires energy between meals, hormones signal the fat cells to break down triglycerides and release fatty acids to be burned for energy.

Problems can develop when too many triglycerides circulate in the blood. People who carry more weight in their abdomen than on their hips and thighs are more likely to have elevated triglyceride levels than people who carry more weight on their hips and thighs. The reason for this is that fat cells in the abdominal area release fat (in the form of fatty acids) into the bloodstream faster than do cells in other parts of the body. High fatty acid levels can make the cells less sensitive to insulin, which increases the risk of type 2 diabetes. Also, particles of fat that carry triglycerides absorb or take in cholesterol, lower the level of good HDL cholesterol, and slow the clearance of bad LDL cholesterol from the blood, increasing the risk of heart disease. Levels of triglycerides above 150 mg/dL are considered high.

Many lifestyle habits can affect your triglyceride levels—in both good ways and bad ways. For example, if your triglyceride level is high, drinking alcohol—even small amounts—can cause further increases in blood triglyceride concentrations. Losing weight, reducing your consumption of saturated fat, eliminating trans fats, and boosting your physical activity can all help bring triglycerides down to a healthy level.

However, in addition to diet, heredity plays a significant role in a person's cholesterol level. In some people, the liver does not clear LDL cholesterol from the blood at a normal rate, making them more likely to have elevated blood cholesterol levels. Problems can arise when harmful LDL cholesterol is not cleared from the blood sufficiently by the liver. LDL cholesterol is harmful because it can cause fatty deposits to collect inside artery walls, which can build up and eventually cause heart disease (atherosclerosis), heart attack, or stroke.

If you have a family history of high cholesterol, talk to your doctor about having a cholesterol test. If you find that you have an undesirable cholesterol profile (see page 94), your doctor will recommend steps you can take to improve it, which may include taking cholesterol-lowering medications.

Protein

Your body needs protein to build, maintain, and repair tissues. Protein also carries vitamins and hormones throughout the bloodstream. Proteins are composed of 21 different chemicals known as amino acids. Some are called essential amino acids because your body cannot make them and needs to obtain them from the food you eat. The other group of amino acids, called nonessential amino acids, are produced by the body.

Proteins in foods that come from animal products such as meat, poultry, fish, eggs, and dairy products are considered complete proteins because they provide all of the essential amino acids. However, one of the problems with eating all or most of your protein from animal sources is that these foods can be high in saturated fat and cholesterol, which can cause fatty deposits to build up inside artery walls, increasing the risk of heart disease. Look for low-fat or fat-free dairy products, lean cuts of meat, and white poultry meat without the skin to keep your heart risks low.

Plant-based protein sources—such as whole grains, beans, and nuts—are incomplete proteins and must be combined to provide all the amino acids the body needs. For example, combining beans with rice, or peanut butter with whole grain bread, makes them equivalent to complete proteins. Vegetarians can get an adequate amount of protein by eating combinations of legumes, whole grains, eggs, and dairy products. If your body doesn't get enough protein, it will begin to break down muscle and organ tissue to supply the needed amino acids.

The amount of protein most adults need every day is relatively small—only 0.8 gram of protein per kilogram (2.2 pounds) of body weight. Most adult Americans consume much more protein than they need. It's easy to do, considering that there are 25 to 35 grams of protein in 4 ounces of lean meat, poultry, or fish; 18 grams in a cup of cooked beans or lentils; and 8 grams in a cup of low-fat milk. Protein grams are listed on food labels. The chart at right can help you determine how many grams of protein you may need in a day, based on your weight.

Weight in Pounds	Grams of Protein Per Day
140	51
150	55
160	59
170	62
180	65
190	69
200	73
210	76
220	80
230	84
240	87
250	91

Vitamins and Minerals

Vitamins and minerals are essential for healthy functioning of the body. Except for vitamin D, which your skin manufactures when it is exposed to sunlight, these essential nutrients are not produced by the body, so you must get them from the food you eat. People can become deficient in vitamin D from lack of exposure to sunlight, especially during the winter months in northern latitudes or if they are elderly and confined to their home.

Although extreme vitamin deficiencies are rare in the United States, many people don't get sufficient vitamins and minerals from their diet. People at risk for vitamin deficiencies include older people (who tend to eat less), women who are pregnant or breast-feeding, people on very-low-calorie weight-loss diets, vegetarians who avoid eggs and dairy products (vegans), and people who take medications that block the absorption of vitamins and minerals. Although it's best to get nutrients from food, many doctors recommend that people take a daily multivitamin and mineral supplement to help ensure an adequate intake.

However, although taking a daily multivitamin may be helpful, consuming megadoses of certain vitamins or minerals can be harmful. Taking vitamin supplements should never be a substitute for eating a healthy diet because food supplies other important nutrients as well, including fiber, essential fatty acids, and protein.

Vitamins and Minerals

The best way to get the vitamins and minerals your body needs is to eat a varied diet, rich in low-fat, high-fiber vegetables, fruits, legumes, and whole grains. The table below describes the health benefits of the most important vitamins and minerals and some of the foods that contain these nutrients.

Vitamins are either fat soluble or water soluble. Fat-soluble vitamins are found in fats and oils in foods and are stored in body fat. Water-soluble vitamins dissolve in water and mix in the blood. Your body stores only small amounts of water-soluble vitamins (the excess is eliminated in urine). Some vitamins are antioxidants, which protect against damage to cells by free radicals (molecules formed by normal cell processes). Antioxidants can help protect against aging and disease, including type 2 diabetes.

Vitamin or Mineral	Good Sources	Health Benefits
FAT-SOLUBLE VITAMINS		
Vitamin A	Fortified milk, eggs, cheese, butter, liver, cod and halibut, fish oil	Antioxidant; essential for growth and development; maintains healthy vision, skin, and mucous membranes
Vitamin D	Fortified milk, salmon, mackerel,	Builds bones and teeth; helps the body absorb and use calcium
Vitamin E	Vegetable oils, whole grains, wheat germ, nuts, green leafy vegetables	Antioxidant; anti-inflammatory; helps form blood cells, muscles, and lung and nerve tissue; boosts the immune system
Vitamin K	Dark green leafy vegetables, liver, egg yolks	Essential for blood clotting
Beta carotene	Orange and deep yellow vegetables and fruits (carrots, sweet potatoes, winter squash, cantaloupe, pumpkins, mangoes); the body converts beta carotene in these vegetables and fruits into vitamin A	Antioxidant; used by the body to make vitamin A
WATER-SOLUBLE VITAMINS		
Vitamin C	Citrus fruits, some vegetables (tomatoes, bell peppers), leafy green vegetables	Antioxidant; keeps bones, teeth, and skin healthy; helps wounds heal
Thiamin (vitamin B1)	Whole-grain and fortified-grain products, pork, peas	Helps convert food into energy
Riboflavin (vitamin B2)	Meats, fish, whole-grain and fortified-grain products, milk products, dark green vegetables	Helps in energy production and other body processes; helps maintain healthy eyes, skin, and nerve function
Niacin (vitamin B3)	Whole-grain and fortified-grain products, milk products, pork, poultry, fish, nuts, broccoli	Helps convert food into energy, and maintain brain function

Vitamin or Mineral	Good Sources	Health Benefits
Vitamin B6	Fortified grains, whole-wheat products, meat, fish, nuts, green beans, bananas, potatoes	Helps produce essential proteins and convert protein into energy
Vitamin B12	Dairy products, eggs, liver, animal products	Helps convert carbohydrates into energy, form red blood cells, maintain the central nervous system, and make amino acids
Folic acid (folate)	Orange juice; dark green leafy vegetables; fruits; dried beans, lentils, and peas; liver	Helps prevent birth defects and form red blood cells, and may lower homocystein in the blood

MINERALS

Calcium	Dairy products, fortified orange juice, fortified-grain products, fortified soy milk, legumes, canned fish (with bones), dark green leafy vegetables	Builds bones and teeth and maintains bone strength; helps control blood pressure; important in muscle function
Chromium	Whole grains, bran cereals, green beans, broccoli, spices, processed meats	Enhances the effects of the hormone insulin in converting sugar, protein, and fat into energy
Copper	Oysters, nuts, legumes, whole grains, vegetables, red meat	Essential for making hemoglobin; helps body absorb and use iron; helps in energy production; keeps bones, blood, and nerves healthy
Iron	Meat, whole-grain and fortified-grain products, poultry, fish, dried beans, nuts, dried fruits	Helps in the production of red blood cells; helps carry oxygen in the bloodstream and deliver it to muscles
Magnesium	Leafy green vegetables, nuts, whole grains, legumes, dairy products, fish, meat, poultry	Essential for healthy nerve and muscle function and for bone formation; helps prevent irregular heartbeat; helps lower blood pressure
Phosphorus	Meat, dairy products, poultry, fish	Builds strong bones and teeth; promotes activity of genes and cells; helps produce and store energy
Potassium	Bananas, oranges, and other fruits; starchy vegetables; nuts and seeds	Helps maintain balance of body fluids, transmit nerve signals, produce energy, lower blood pressure, and prevent irregular heartbeat
Selenium	Fish, meat, Brazil nuts	Antioxidant; essential for healthy heart and immune system
Sodium	Table salt, processed foods, canned soups	Helps maintain normal blood pressure, balance body fluids, and transmit nerve signals
Zinc	Fortified-grain products, shellfish, meat, legumes, nuts, eggs, yogurt	Promotes cell reproduction, growth and development, the immune response, nervous system function, reproduction, and wound healing

Eat Your Antioxidants

Antioxidants are molecules that fight potentially cell-damaging molecules called free radicals, which are by-products of normal cell processes in the body. Free radicals are also produced when blood sugar is elevated and are thought to be a factor in the development of type 2 diabetes. Excessive exposure to sunlight and other forms of radiation is another source of free-radical production in the body.

Although free radicals are essential to life, they become harmful when they outnumber antioxidants in the body. By keeping free radicals in check, antioxidants are thought to not only promote good health, but also help to prevent many of the most common chronic diseases (including type 2 diabetes) and, possibly, to slow the aging process. Some vitamins and minerals are antioxidants. Examples of antioxidant vitamins are vitamins C, E, and beta carotene (a form of vitamin A). The minerals selenium, magnesium, copper, and zinc are also considered antioxidants.

In addition to antioxidants, fruits and vegetables have lots of protective vitamins and phytochemicals. Lycopene, for example, is a phytochemical found in tomatoes, pink grapefruit, and watermelon that has been shown to lower the risk of prostate cancer and heart disease. Some foods contain many different antioxidants in especially high amounts. These extra-healthy foods include blueberries and other berries, spinach, carrots, cantaloupe, winter squash, broccoli and other cruciferous vegetables, apricots, citrus fruits, nuts, and seeds. Think color: in general, the more colorful the fruit or vegetable, the more nutrients it provides.

Because of the strong evidence for the disease-lowering, health-promoting benefits of eating lots of fruits and vegetables, the newest Dietary Guidelines for Americans (see page 116) call for everyone to try to eat 5 to 13 servings of fruits and vegetables every day. This is especially important if you are at risk of developing type 2 diabetes. Eating a good amount of fruits and vegetables every day can also reduce your risk of heart disease and stroke.

Thirteen servings a day sounds like a lot, but it's easier to achieve than you think, especially when you are aware of what a serving actually is (see below). You can get 3 servings of fruit at breakfast by having ½ cup of blueberries, a slice of melon, and 6 ounces of low-sodium vegetable juice. Add a serving for a mid-morning snack with a medium apple, ¼ cup of raisins, or ½ cup of cut-up carrots or celery, and you've already had 4 servings before lunch. Get 3 servings at lunch with 3 cups of salad. Have a medium banana for dessert and an orange for an afternoon snack, and you're up to 9 servings. For dinner, have 2 servings of vegetables, a salad, and fruit for dessert and you've got your 13 servings of fruits and veggies. Most important, you've given yourself a healthy dose of protective antioxidants.

What Counts as a Serving?

The servings of fruits and vegetables needed to maintain good health are relatively small, making it easier than you think to consume 10 to 13 servings a day. One serving translates into:

- 1 medium-sized piece of fruit
- ½ cup cut-up fresh or canned fruit
- 1 cup raw leafy vegetables or salad

- ½ cup cooked or canned vegetables
- ¾ cup (6 ounces) vegetable juice
- ½ cup cooked or canned beans, peas, or lentils
- ¾ cup (6 ounces) 100 percent fruit juice (but drink only in moderation)
- ¼ cup dried fruit, such as raisins (but eat only in moderation)

Salt and High Blood Pressure

Table salt, or sodium chloride, is an essential nutrient, needed to balance water and minerals in the body and to aid the function of nerves and muscles. But problems can arise when you consume too much salt. Excess salt makes the body retain water, which raises blood volume and can raise blood pressure, especially in people who are overweight or sensitive to the effects of sodium.

Many people who are at risk for type 2 diabetes are also at risk for high blood pressure (see page 93), or hypertension, because both conditions tend to develop with weight gain and advancing age. Like type 2 diabetes, hypertension is considered a silent disease because it seldom causes symptoms in the early stages. However, even without causing symptoms, both conditions can damage tissues throughout the body. Have your blood pressure checked at each doctor visit. If your blood pressure is higher than 120/80 mm Hg (high blood pressure is a reading above 140/90), you have prehypertension, which puts you at high risk of developing hypertension. Your doctor will recommend steps you can take to lower your blood pressure, including reducing your consumption of salt.

Because sodium is plentiful in so many foods on grocery store shelves, most Americans eat three to five times as much sodium as their body needs. The majority of the salt we eat comes from processed and fast foods, not the salt shaker. It's not easy to avoid salty foods and restrict your salt intake. The first step is to carefully check food labels for sodium content, especially on packaged and canned foods. Choose those that indicate that they are low sodium, reduced sodium, sodium-free, or no salt added. Look for less than 140 milligrams of sodium per serving.

Watch out for notoriously high-sodium foods such as canned soups, the flavor packets in rice and pasta, sandwich meats and sausages, smoked meats and fish, and snack foods such as chips. And be on the

Three Important Minerals

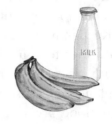

If you have high blood pressure, increasing your consumption of foods containing the minerals calcium, potassium, and magnesium can help improve your blood pressure. Calcium has been shown to lower blood pressure. To achieve this beneficial effect, you need to consume 1,000 to 1,500 milligrams of calcium each day. Potassium balances sodium in the body, helping to control blood pressure and reduce the risk of stroke. Magnesium helps lower blood pressure.

Calcium-rich foods include dairy products (even those that are low-fat and fat-free) and green leafy vegetables. Potassium-rich foods include many fruits, vegetables, dairy foods, and fish. The best sources of magnesium are whole grains, green leafy vegetables, nuts, seeds, and legumes.

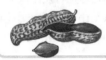

You can easily boost your intake of these key minerals by eating 5 to 13 servings of fruit and vegetables each day and consuming 3 servings of fat-free milk or yogurt daily.

lookout for the following food additives on labels because they contain some forms of salt: sodium nitrate, sodium benzoate, and monosodium glutamate (MSG). Other, more hidden sources of sodium include some over-the-counter medications, club soda, baking powder, baking soda, and many seasonings such as chili powder and soy sauce.

We are not born with a taste for salt—we acquire it over time from eating salty foods. You may find it difficult at first to go low-sodium, but once you readjust your taste buds to savor flavors other than salt, you will learn not to miss it. Experiment with sodium-free flavorings, including herbs and spices, lemon and lime juices, and garlic and onion powders. Add salt-free seasoning blends to soups, stews, and casseroles.

Alcohol and Diabetes

It has been known for years that people who drink alcohol in moderation have a lower risk of heart disease than people who don't drink at all. However, doctors do not recommend that people take up drinking as a way to prevent heart disease. It also looks as if moderate alcohol consumption may reduce the risk of type 2 diabetes. But the key is moderation. Moderate drinking is defined as up to two drinks a day for men and one drink a day for women. A drink is generally considered to be 12 ounces of beer, 5 ounces of wine, or 1.5 ounces of liquor, each of which contains 15 grams of alcohol and 105 calories.

Keep in mind that consuming excessive amounts of alcohol adds lots of calories to your diet, which can lead to weight gain and associated health risks, including heart disease and type 2 diabetes. Excessive drinking can cause other serious health problems as well, including high blood pressure, liver damage, and inflammation of the pancreas. Excessive alcohol use can also cause vitamin deficiencies and malnutrition. Drinking during pregnancy can cause a group of birth defects called fetal alcohol syndrome, which is the most common preventable cause of mental retardation in the United States.

Alcohol affects women faster than it does men because women are generally smaller than men. Also, the female hormone estrogen delays the speed at which the liver processes alcohol, so women who drink large amounts of alcohol tend to get intoxicated faster and incur liver damage earlier than men who drink the same amounts.

The most sensible advice: if you don't drink now, don't start. If you drink, limit your consumption to one drink a day if you're a woman and two drinks a day if you're a man.

Healthy Eating for the Whole Family

You can help family members be healthy by serving nutritious foods and instilling healthy eating habits in your children that they can follow throughout their life. It may not be easy to schedule family meals when you work and your kids have after-school activities, but eating together is one of the most important things you can do to promote good health habits in your household. Family meals are not only comforting and predictable for children, but they also give you a chance to introduce new foods and find out which foods your children like.

Serve a variety of foods, with an emphasis on vegetables, fruits, and whole grains. Set a good example by eating healthfully yourself. Children who regularly have meals with their parents are less likely to snack on unwholesome foods and are more likely to eat fruits and vegetables. They are also less likely to be overweight. An additional benefit: they are less likely than their peers who don't share family meals to engage in unhealthy behaviors such as smoking or using alcohol or illegal drugs.

Stock the Kitchen with Healthy Foods

Having nutritious ingredients on hand allows you to pull together healthy meals quickly and easily. Stock plenty of canned and frozen fruits and vegetables (those without added sugars and salt). Keep an extra loaf of whole-grain, high-fiber bread in the freezer. Read food labels carefully, especially noting the type of fat in the food (limit foods with saturated fats and avoid foods with trans fats), the total fat grams per serving (look for less than 3 grams), the amount of sodium (look for less than 140 milligrams), and the fiber content (look for more than 3 grams). Stay away from processed and commercially packaged convenience foods because they are often high in sodium and fat. Here's a list of healthy foods to have in your pantry:

Grains and Beans

- Whole-grain, high-fiber breads
- A variety of dried pastas (including whole-wheat or half-wheat pastas, which provide more fiber than white pastas)
- Rice—especially brown and wild rice
- Whole grains—such as barley, cornmeal, bulgur, couscous, and oats
- Whole-grain, high-fiber cereals (avoid instant and packaged cereals that are low in fiber and high in sugar, salt, and trans fats)
- Dried and canned legumes—such as lentils, kidney and black beans, black-eyed peas, and chickpeas

Vegetables

- Vegetables that enhance flavor—such as onions, garlic, and shallots
- A variety of frozen and low-sodium canned vegetables—such as broccoli, spinach, beans, and cauliflower
- Low-sodium canned tomatoes
- Low-sodium tomato and vegetable cocktail juices
- Dried and low-sodium canned mushrooms

Fruits

- Frozen berries
- Fruits canned in water or natural juices (but consume only in moderate amounts)

- Bottled, canned, and frozen fruit juices (but drink only in moderate amounts)
- Dried fruit (but eat only in small amounts)

Dairy Foods

- Fat-free milk—fresh, dried, and canned
- Reduced-fat cheeses (kept in the freezer)
- Fat-free or low-fat refrigerated cheeses (including cottage cheese) and fat-free and sugar-free yogurt

Meat, Poultry, Fish, Eggs, and Nuts

- Poultry, lean pork, lean beef, and fish (kept in the freezer)
- Canned tuna, salmon, and sardines, packed in water
- Frozen egg substitute
- Natural, nonhydrogenated peanut butter that is low in sugar and salt
- A variety of nuts (the healthiest are raw, without added salt or sugar)

Fats, Oils, and Sweets

- Cooking oils, especially olive oil and canola oil
- Nonstick cooking oil spray
- Tub or liquid margarine without trans fats and margarine with plant sterols or stanols
- White and brown sugar, honey, and artificial sweetener, if desired

Additional Ingredients

- A variety of spices
- A variety of vinegars
- A variety of mustards (without added sugars)
- Pickles, olives, and condiments (without added sugars)
- Whole-grain flours, vanilla and other extracts, and other ingredients for baking
- Canned low-sodium, fat-free broths

Adding Flavor to Foods

It's easier than you think to enhance the flavor of foods without adding a lot of unhealthy fat or salt. Experiment with dried herbs and spices to heighten the taste and aroma of your favorite foods. Try these popular flavor enhancers:

- **Olive Oil**   Rich in healthy monounsaturated fats, olive oil also provides an antioxidant boost. Extra-virgin olive oil, which comes from the first pressing of the olives, is the finest quality, but any type imparts the oil's characteristic flavor. Use olive oil for cooking, on salads, and as a dip for bread. You can find flavored varieties in many stores. Store the oil in a cool, dry place. If it smells rancid or musty, throw it away and buy a new bottle.

- **Vinegar**   Stock a variety of vinegars to use in salads and marinades and to sprinkle on veggies. A tablespoon of balsamic or red wine vinegar in stews and soups adds a punch of flavor. Always keep a variety of vinegars, along with cooking wines, to add interest to dishes.

Healthy Food Substitutions

When you cut fat from your meals, you also cut calories, but that doesn't mean you have to give up taste. Use the following healthy food substitutions to make your meals nutritious, lower in calories and fat, and still delicious and satisfying.

Instead of . . .	Use . . .
Full-fat or 2% milk	Fat-free milk
Full-fat yogurt	Low-fat or fat-free yogurt
Full-fat or light ice cream	Sherbet or low-fat or fat-free frozen yogurt or ice cream
Regular cheese	Low-fat or fat-free cheese (but check the sodium content, which is often high)
Sour cream	Fat-free sour cream or low-fat yogurt
Whipped cream	Whipped evaporated skim milk
Cream cheese	Fat-free or light (Neufchâtel) cream cheese
Mayonnaise or salad dressing	Reduced-fat or low-fat mayonnaise or salad dressing
Salt	Herbs, spices, lemon and lime juices, flavored vinegar
Canned broth or bouillon	Fat-free, reduced-sodium broth
1 whole egg	2 egg whites
White flour	Whole-wheat flour (increase the recipe's liquids)
White cake flour	Whole-wheat pastry flour (increase the recipe's liquids)
White pasta	Whole-grain pasta
White rice	Brown rice

How to Read Food Labels

The Nutrition Facts panel is the part of a food package label that lists the serving size, the number of servings in the package, the number of calories in a serving, and the number of grams and the percentage of daily values (which are the same as the recommended daily allowances) of many important nutrients—including fat, carbohydrate, cholesterol, fiber, and sodium.

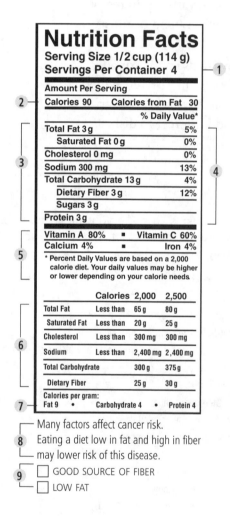

Many factors affect cancer risk. Eating a diet low in fat and high in fiber may lower risk of this disease.

☐ GOOD SOURCE OF FIBER
☐ LOW FAT

What Food Labels Can Tell You

1. To make it easy to compare different brands of the same food, all serving sizes of the food are required to be the same.
2. This line shows the total calories in one serving and how many calories from fat are contained in the serving.
3. This section displays the amounts of different nutrients in one serving so you can easily compare the nutrient content of similar products and add up the total amounts of a given nutrient that you eat in a day.
4. The percentage of daily values is indicated for most of the nutrients. (No daily values have been set for protein and sugar.) Percentages of daily values are based on a diet of 2,000 calories per day.
5. This area shows the percentage of daily values for vitamins A and C and the minerals iron and calcium.
6. This section helps you calculate your daily allowance of various fats, sodium, carbohydrates, and fiber for both a 2,000- and a 2,500-calorie-per-day diet.
7. The number of calories in 1 gram of fat, carbohydrate, and protein are shown here.
8. The federal government has approved the use of certain health claims on packaged foods. Examples include:
   - A diet low in fat and rich in fruits and vegetables may reduce your risk of some cancers.
   - A diet rich in fruits, vegetables, and grains may reduce the risk of heart disease.
   - A low intake of calcium is one risk factor for osteoporosis.
9. Terms such as "low," "high," and "free" on food labels must meet strict definitions. For example, a food described as "very low sodium" must have no more than 35 milligrams of sodium for every 50 grams of food.

- **Hard Cheeses** Keep a block of strongly flavored hard cheese in the refrigerator and grate a small amount over cooked pasta, chili, and other dishes for added taste. Good choices are Parmesan and Romano.
- **Broths** Chicken, beef, and vegetable broths add a lot of flavor to soups, tomato sauces, and Asian dishes. Cook rice, couscous, and other whole grains with broth instead of water. But make sure the broth you use is low in sodium and fat-free. You can also make your own broth and freeze it in usable quantities.
- **Nuts** A handful of chopped or ground (unsalted) nuts goes a long way when it comes to both flavor and health. Nuts increase the protein content of a meal and contain heart-healthy unsaturated fat. Toss some nuts into a salad, a pasta dish, a fish entrée, or a vegetable side dish.
- **Tomatoes** Cooked tomatoes are especially nutritious because they contain the powerful cancer-fighting antioxidant lycopene. Canned cooked tomatoes are convenient and come in many varieties, already flavored with oregano, olive oil, hot peppers, garlic, and onions—and already chopped.
- **Garlic** With its heart-healthy nutrients, fresh garlic is a must for every kitchen. Garlic brings out the best flavors of any cuisine. Mince a couple of cloves and sauté them quickly—1 minute or less for the best taste.
- **Salsa** This Mexican dip doesn't have to be spicy to perk up the taste of foods as varied as a baked potato, an omelet, or a bean burrito. In fact, you can substitute it for almost any high-fat sauce.

Nutritious Snacks

Americans' favorite snack foods tend to be high in trans fats and saturated fat, salt, and sugar, but you don't have to choose these. You can easily make your snacks an additional source of nutrients. The first—and most important—step is to resist the temptation to buy the familiar favorites when you're at the store. (Hint: this is easier to do if you go grocery shopping on a full stomach.) If you don't have sugary soft drinks, doughnuts, cupcakes, or chips at home, you and your family won't reach for them when you're hungry. Here are some suggestions for healthy munching:

- Cut-up raw vegetables
- Fresh fruit, whole or cut up
- Low-fat mozzarella cheese sticks
- Peanut butter on whole-grain graham crackers
- Unsalted nuts or seeds
- Air-popped or low-fat microwave popcorn (look for brands that are low in sodium and without hydrogenated oils or trans fats)
- A fruit-and-yogurt smoothie
- Applesauce
- Sliced turkey rolled up in a whole-wheat tortilla

Read labels when you shop to make sure the snack foods you buy don't contain partially hydrogenated oils, a major source of harmful trans fats. Check all peanut butter, crackers, tortillas, and breads for trans fats. Buy only low- or reduced-sodium and whole-grain items. You may have to supplement your major grocery shopping with an occasional trip to a health food store to find a more varied selection of nutritious choices.

5

Exercise Your Way to Better Health

Like a sensible diet, exercise is essential for good health. Millions of Americans who are at increased risk for type 2 diabetes can sharply lower their chances of developing the disorder by becoming more physically active. When combined with a healthy diet and weight loss, exercise is a safe and effective way to prevent diabetes. In fact, exercise, when combined with weight loss, has been found to work at least as well as the diabetes medication metformin (see page 132)—possibly even better—in reducing type 2 diabetes risk.

Physical activity prevents or delays the development of diabetes in two important ways. Exercise helps cells use the circulating blood sugar they need for energy production by making the cells more sensitive to the hormone insulin, even if you don't also lose weight. But a weight loss of just a few pounds can improve your insulin sensitivity even more. Here are some ways exercise reduces your risk of type 2 diabetes as well as high blood pressure, heart attack, and stroke:

- Lowers blood glucose level
- Reduces blood pressure
- Lowers bad LDL cholesterol and raises good HDL cholesterol levels
- Strengthens the heart muscle
- Reduces body fat

Exercise also reduces your risk of other common disorders, including the bone-thinning condition osteoporosis and some cancers. Here's how exercise improves your health in other ways:

- Builds strong muscles, bones, and joints
- Enhances your flexibility and balance
- Lessens your risk of falling
- Relieves arthritis pain
- Improves your mood
- Reduces stress
- Makes you look and feel better
- Improves your sleep

Any amount of exercise is better than none, but the federal government, alarmed by the increasing weight of Americans, has established new guidelines for exercise. The guidelines recommend at least 30 minutes of moderate-intensity physical activity every day to reduce the risk of chronic diseases such as type 2 diabetes and heart disease. The guidelines also call for 60 minutes of moderate to vigorous physical activity most days to prevent weight gain, and 60 to 90 minutes of daily physical activity to lose weight.

If you have been sedentary for a while, start slowly and work up to 30 minutes a day at a pace that is comfortable for you. If you can't sustain physical activity for 30 minutes, or feel that you are just too busy to carve that much time out of your day for exercise, accumulate activity over the course of the day in 10- or 15-minute intervals. The exercise will add up and the health benefits will be the same. Try to eventually work up to 60 to 90 minutes of exercise most days of the week.

Exercise doesn't necessarily have to be vigorous to provide health benefits. Even moderate exercise such as walking can substantially reduce your risk of developing type 2 diabetes. Many people who are at risk for type 2 diabetes are overweight, and this excess weight places a lot of stress on the muscles and joints, especially those in the hips, knees, and ankles. If you are overweight, try lower-impact activities such as walking or swimming when you begin your exercise program. Later, when you're better conditioned and stronger, try more vigorous activities such as aerobic classes, jogging, or biking.

If you are overweight, you may be susceptible to discomfort or pain when you exercise. Injuries, such as strains and sprains, are more likely to occur in overweight people. For this reason, start out slowly when you're beginning an exercise program. Make sure you wear socks and sturdy, comfortable shoes that are right for the activity (see page 81).

Types of Exercise

There are three main types of exercise—aerobic, strength training, and flexibility—and each provides health benefits. Aerobic activities such as brisk walking, jogging, and bicycling make your heart work harder and more efficiently. Strength-training exercises such as push-ups and weight-lifting build strong muscles and bones. Flexibility exercises such as yoga and stretching increase the joints' range of motion.

Aerobic and strength-training exercises are especially effective in preventing type 2 diabetes. Aerobic exercise makes your cells more sensitive to insulin and, by burning calories and aiding weight loss, can help keep blood glucose levels from rising. Strength training decreases body fat by raising metabolism and building muscle, which burns more calories than fat. Flexibility exercises are important because they help maintain balance and prevent joint stiffness. They also reduce the risk of falls, which can result in fractured or broken bones. To become fit, you need to incorporate all three types of exercise into your routine.

Aerobic Exercise

Continuous, repetitive, and prolonged movements that use the large muscles of the arms and legs define aerobic exercise. Examples of aerobic exercise include brisk walking, climbing stairs, hiking, jogging, swimming, doing water aerobics, riding a bike, rowing, dancing, and cross-country skiing. Aerobic exercises in which your bones support your weight, such as walking and jogging, strengthen your bones and reduce the risk of the bone-thinning disorder osteoporosis. Non-weight-bearing exercises such as swimming and riding a bike do not. However, low-impact exercises such as these don't put as much stress on the joints as weight-bearing exercises do.

Regardless of the activity, however, all aerobic exercise makes your cardiovascular system stronger, reducing your risk of heart disease and high blood pressure. Regular aerobic exercise also increases your endurance, enabling you to walk, bike, or swim farther and for a longer time.

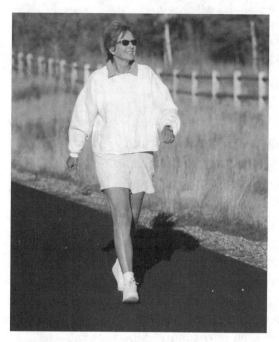

Aerobic Exercise

Walking is the form of exercise doctors recommend most. People who walk at least an hour a day are much less likely than inactive people to develop type 2 diabetes, high blood pressure, or heart disease, or to have a heart attack or a stroke.

Activities done at a moderate intensity are best, at least initially, because you can sustain them longer and you're less likely to get discouraged. At a moderate pace, you should find it a little harder to talk but still be able to hold a conversation. In fact, being able to carry on a conversation is a good gauge of how vigorously you are exercising. If you cannot speak, you are exercising too intensely. If you have no trouble talking at all, you may be going at too leisurely a pace. Try to exercise hard enough to reach your target heart rate (see page 77) for at least 20 minutes each session.

Strength-Building Exercises

Strength training, also known as strength conditioning or resistance training, refers to repeated bouts of intense activity using free weights or circuit-type weight machines that force the body's muscles to work against an outside weight. Exercises without weights—such as sit-ups, pull-ups, push-ups, lunges, and leg lifts—are also considered strength conditioning because they make your muscles work against the weight of your body.

Strength-training exercises make you fit by developing stronger bones, muscles, and joints. They also help you burn extra calories because muscle burns more calories than fat. But the good news for people at risk for diabetes is that strength training can help make your cells more sensitive to insulin and enable muscle cells to absorb sugar from the blood more efficiently.

Just as important, weight training is good for the heart, because people who are at risk for type 2 diabetes are also at increased risk for heart disease. Without exercise, many of us tend to gain fat and lose muscle as we age. Resistance training helps you lose body fat and rebuild muscle. In addition, weight training lowers the risk of falling, an especially important consideration for older people.

You can easily and conveniently perform strength-training exercises

Strengthening Exercises

Strength-conditioning exercise reduces your risk of type 2 diabetes by making your cells more sensitive to insulin and more efficient at taking in glucose from the blood. Like aerobic exercise, strengthening exercise is beneficial for your heart and can help you lose weight (because muscles burn more calories than fat). These exercises build muscle by forcing the muscles to work against the weight of your body. It's a good idea to alternate strength-building exercises with aerobic exercise. Try to do the following exercises three or four times a week.

Modified Push-up

Get on your hands and knees on the floor and shift your weight forward, with your hands aligned under your shoulders and your feet raised off the floor (*top*). Bending your elbows, lower your body from the knees up until your chest almost touches the floor, keeping your hands in the same position on the floor and using your abdominal muscles to keep your back straight (*bottom*). Still keeping your back straight, push up until your arms are almost straight (but not locked) at the elbows. Repeat as many times as you can without straining. (For an extra challenge, try holding each position for a few seconds.)

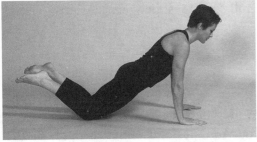

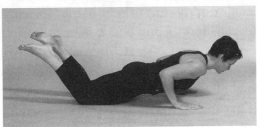

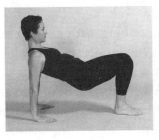

Triceps Press

Sit on the floor with your knees bent at a 45-degree angle, your feet flat on the floor, hip-distance apart, and your hands on the floor behind you, fingertips pointing forward. Lift your hips off the floor (left). Bending at the elbows, lower your bottom until it almost touches the floor (right), hold for a count of 5, and straighten the arms, returning to your starting hips-up position. Do 10 sets.

Abdominal Curl

Lie on your back with your knees bent and your arms holding the backs of your thighs. Press the small of your back into the floor as you lift your head and upper body until most of your upper back is off the floor. Hold for a count of 2. Lower your body to the floor, keeping the small of your back pressed to the floor (to work your abdominal muscles and avoid straining your back). As your strength increases, increase the number of repetitions. A more difficult way to do sit-ups is with your arms over your chest, hands on the shoulders, or with your hands placed lightly behind your neck.

at home with inexpensive, lightweight dumbbells. You can also improvise weights with cans of soup or books. Do a few sets of lifts whenever you find yourself sitting in front of the TV, or do the strengthening exercises shown on page 73.

Using weight machines is a more efficient way to weight train because you can target specific muscle groups and choose the exact amount of weight to work against. Doctors suggest doing strength-training exercises two or three days a week, performing 8 to 10 repetitions of each exercise. Take a full day of rest between sessions to let your muscles rest and recover.

Flexibility Exercises

If you are relatively inactive or sedentary as you get older, you will become less able to move your muscles and joints through their full range of motion. This reduced flexibility can make it harder for you to carry out everyday tasks and can boost your chances of falling and breaking a bone. Flexibility exercises, such as stretching, can help maintain movement in your joints and protect your muscles from injury as you go about your daily routine. Flexibility exercises also help you keep your balance when walking or getting up from a sitting position. Added benefits of flexibility exercises are improved circulation and relief of muscle tension. These exercises may also help you avoid injury if you stretch before doing an aerobic exercise such as walking.

Taking yoga or Pilates classes or stretching along with a video are excellent ways to extend and tone your muscles and limber up your joints. Doing simple stretches of your arms, back, and legs in the morning are also good ways to increase your flexibility. The key muscles to stretch are the hamstrings in the backs of your thighs and the muscles in the lower back and shoulders. Follow these recommendations for getting the most benefit our of your stretching and reducing the risk of injury:

- If you feel pain, ease up on your stretch. Pain is a sign that you have extended too far.
- Stretch slowly and smoothly to avoid muscle injury. Don't bounce or jerk.
- Stretch as far as you comfortably can and hold your stretch for 30 seconds to give your muscles and joints the full benefits of the stretch.

Exercises That Increase Flexibility

Increased flexibility improves your ability to perform everyday activities, protects your muscles against pulls and tears, and helps relieve arthritis pain. It's important to do stretches gently and slowly—don't bounce. Do each stretch three times for maximum benefit.

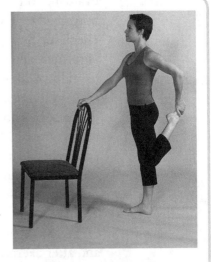

Hip Flexor/Quadriceps Stretch

Standing up, hold on to a sturdy chair back, a counter, or a railing with one hand. Bend one leg and, with the hand on that side, pull your foot up gently behind you, keeping your abdominal muscles pulled in and your knees close together. Maintain the position for at least 30 seconds. Repeat with the other leg.

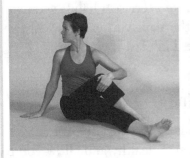

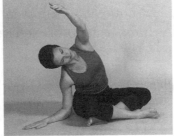

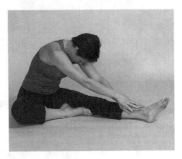

Back Twist

Sit up with your legs out in front of you on the floor. Cross one leg over the other with your knee bent and foot flat on the floor. Keeping your back straight and buttocks on the floor, take hold of the bent knee with the opposite hand and gently turn to the bent-knee side, rotating your hips and looking over your shoulder. Maintain the stretch for at least 30 seconds. Repeat on the other side.

Side Stretch

Sit cross-legged on the floor. Inhale, raise one arm to the ceiling, and, exhaling, bend from the waist to the opposite side, sliding the other hand along the floor and keeping your buttocks on the floor. Maintain the stretch for at least 30 seconds. Inhale as you return to center, dropping your raised arm and lifting the other arm and repeating the bend to the other side.

Hamstring Stretch

Sit with one leg extended in front of you and the other leg bent. Reach forward with both hands along your extended leg as far as it feels comfortable. Bend from your hips, keeping your back straight. Maintain the position for at least 30 seconds. Repeat with the other leg.

Beginning an Exercise Program

If you have one or more risk factors for type 2 diabetes or have another chronic health problem—such as obesity, high blood pressure, or heart disease—you should have a complete physical examination by your doctor before beginning an exercise regimen. Your doctor will want to evaluate you for conditions that could be made worse by exercise. You may need to have an electrocardiogram and an exercise treadmill test to check for heart problems, especially if you want to participate in more vigorous exercise.

Talk with your doctor about the kind of activities that are best for you. Walking is an excellent form of exercise recommended by most doctors, but no matter what activity you choose, start slowly and gradually increase the level of intensity and length of time to increase your endurance. Aim for a gradual buildup of physical activity from a minimum of 30 minutes a day to 60 to 90 minutes every day. If you can't carve out a 30-minute block of time, exercise in two 15-minute sessions or three 10-minute sessions to reach your goal.

Wear the proper footwear (see page 81). Drink some water before and after exercising—this is especially important when you're exercising outdoors in the heat. Most important, make exercise a habit—you will find that you feel noticeably better on the days you exercise. Always keep in mind that the benefits of exercise don't last if you stop.

Fitting Exercise into Your Daily Routine

How can someone as busy as you fit exercise into your life? You have to make it a priority. Exercise will help you stay healthy and allow you to enjoy life—and it may even help you live longer. If you have been inactive for a long time, motivate yourself to get moving. Instead of trying to squeeze exercise into your hectic day, try planning your day around your 30 to 60 minutes of exercise each day. Just as smart investors pay themselves first by setting savings aside before paying the bills, you can pay yourself first by making physical activity a priority time—time that will pay big dividends in improved health.

Once you have set aside the time, set goals; setting and achieving small goals is an excellent way to keep yourself motivated. For example, set a goal of walking or jogging half a mile and then celebrate your success when you reach the goal. Track your progress in a log so you can see your improvement. Alternate among a variety of activities so you don't get bored. Walk one day, swim the next, and exercise to a video on another day. Tell your family and friends about your commitment to regular exercise and encourage them to support you—and join you.

Your Target Heart Rate

A good way of pacing yourself when you exercise is to measure your target heart rate every so often. To calculate your target heart rate, you simply take your pulse periodically while you exercise and see if it stays in a range that is 50 to 75 percent of your maximum heart rate. If your pulse is under 50 percent, exercise a little more vigorously to bring it up. If it is more than 75 percent of your maximum heart rate, slow down a little until your pulse reaches the optimal range. Your maximum and target heart rates depend on your age. To find your maximum heart rate, subtract your age from 220. The chart below shows estimated target heart rates for different ages. Look for the age closest to yours and read across to find your maximum heart rate and your target heart rate range.

FIND YOUR TARGET

Age	Target Heart Rate Range (50–75% of maximum)	Maximum Heart Rate (100%)
20 years	100–150 beats per minute	200 beats per minute
25 years	98–146 beats per minute	195 beats per minute
30 years	95–142 beats per minute	190 beats per minute
35 years	93–138 beats per minute	185 beats per minute
40 years	90–135 beats per minute	180 beats per minute
45 years	88–131 beats per minute	175 beats per minute
50 years	85–127 beats per minute	170 beats per minute
55 years	83–123 beats per minute	165 beats per minute
60 years	80–120 beats per minute	160 beats per minute
65 years	78–116 beats per minute	155 beats per minute
70 years	75–113 beats per minute	150 beats per minute

If you are just starting out on an exercise program, try to reach the lower end (50 percent) of your target zone during the first few weeks. As you get more fit, steadily build up to the upper end (75 percent) of the range. Monitoring your target heart rate can help you and your doctor evaluate your progress in your physical activity program and your overall fitness. Medications for high blood pressure can affect heart rate during exercise, so if you are taking a blood pressure medication, ask your doctor what your ideal heart rate range should be.

Find ways to be more active during your daily routine. Here are some simple ways to fit more physical activity into your life:

- Take a brisk walk around the neighborhood with family or friends.
- Take the stairs instead of the elevator or the escalator.
- Park your car farther from the bus stop, grocery store, or other destination.
- Walk around the local shopping mall during bad weather.
- Bike or hike with your family on weekends.
- Stretch, lift weights, ride a stationary bicycle, walk on a treadmill, or do a yoga or Pilates mat routine while watching TV.
- Do your own yard work: garden, rake leaves, and mow the lawn.

Don't be discouraged if you "fall off the wagon" and stop exercising for a time. Begin again on a gradual basis until you get back to your old level and pace.

Preventing and Treating Exercise-Related Injuries

The "no pain, no gain" adage does not apply to exercise. Injuries can occur if you overdo it or fail to take some common-sense precautions when you exercise. Most athletic injuries are overuse injuries that result when muscles and joints are not allowed to rest sufficiently between workouts or when people continue to work out when they experience pain. Being overweight in itself can pose problems because the excess weight puts stress on the joints, especially the knees and hips, and can weaken the muscles in the abdomen and back.

To minimize your risk of injury or other health problems, see your doctor before beginning a regular exercise program if you have been inactive for some time; are over the age of 40; have heart, back, or joint problems; are a smoker; or are overweight or obese. When you first start an exercise program, it's less important to focus on the type of exercise or the amount of exercise and more important to increase the number of days you exercise, even if you start out exercising only one day a week. Your ultimate goal should be to exercise six to seven days a week for at least an hour, or 90 minutes a day if you are trying to lose weight.

Staying Fit as You Age

Exercise is the best way to stop or reverse age-related loss of muscle, and one of the best ways to reduce your risk for type 2 diabetes, heart disease, high blood pressure, and stroke. Strength-building exercises using handheld weights, elastic exercise bands, or weight machines can help you maintain your independence as you age and reduce your risk of falls. Go for frequent walks and do the following exercises at home at least four times a week. You can even do them while you watch TV.

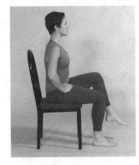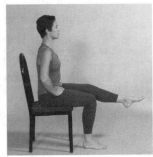

Leg Lift/Leg Extension

Leg lifts help tone the upper leg muscles. Sit with your back straight, knees bent, and both feet flat on the floor. Lift one leg off the floor and extend it in front of you, making sure to pull in your abdominal muscles and center your weight over both hips. Bring the leg slowly back to the starting position. Repeat with the other leg. Do 10 to 15 repetitions with each leg.

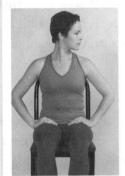

Head Turn/Neck Stretch

Sit with your back straight, feet flat on the floor, and head in an upright position. Turn your head gently and slowly to one side and hold for a count of 5. Turn your head slowly back to the center and then to the other side and hold for 5. Do 5 to 10 times.

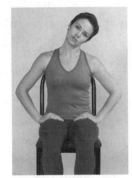

Head Roll/Neck Stretch

Sit with your back straight, feet flat on the floor, and head in an upright position. Roll your head gently and slowly in a circle from one side to the other, flexing your neck at the back of the circle so you are looking up to the point where the front wall meets the ceiling (no higher) and down at your chest at the front of the circle. Repeat the circle from the other direction. Do the sequence 5 to 10 times.

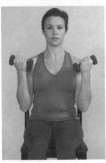

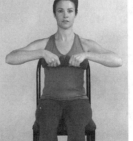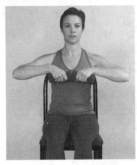

Bicep Curl

Sit with your back straight and feet flat on the floor, hold two small hand weights (begin with 1-pound weights) with your arms bent, the weights up and in toward your shoulders (left). Slowly bring the weights down to the sides of your thighs (right) and then slowly bring them back up to your shoulders. When you can do the sequence 12 times, increase the weights by 1 pound.

Pump-up

Sit with your back straight and feet flat on the floor, holding the ends of two weights together at your chest and keeping your shoulders down and your elbows out (left). Lower the weights slowly to waist level, keeping the ends of the weights together (right). Raise the weights slowly to chest level again. When you can do the sequence 12 times, increase the weights by 1 pound.

Follow the 10-percent rule: increase your activity—such as the distance you walk or run or the size of the weights you use—by no more than 10 percent each week. Strengthen the muscles of your legs for walking or jogging first by riding a bicycle or using a weight machine. Pay attention to your body while you exercise. Slow down or stop for a while if you feel pain in a muscle or joint. After you finish your workout, rest any painful area right away and place an ice bag on it (see RICE, next page).

No matter what type of activity you engage in, try to make time for warm-up and cool-down periods before and after exercising to help reduce your risk of injury. A warm-up can be as simple as 5 minutes of low-intensity aerobic activity that uses the same muscles as those you will use during your workout. For example, walk for 5 minutes before jogging. After you finish exercising, cool down with 5 additional minutes of less intense activity. Doing stretching exercises before and after physical activity will also maintain and increase your overall flexibility, and warming up and cooling down will ease the transition between rest and physical activity.

When working out with exercise equipment, read the instructions carefully or, better yet, ask a qualified trainer to show you how to use it. This will help you get the most benefit out of the equipment and reduce your risk of injury. If you have a treadmill or other exercise equipment at home, make sure it is in good working order.

Always drink plenty of water before, during, and after exercising, especially if you are working out in very dry or humid weather. Unless you are training for a marathon or other endurance competition, you don't need to consume sports drinks with added electrolytes. Most sports drinks contain surprisingly high amounts of sugar.

Don't overexert yourself in extreme temperatures. If the weather is too hot or too cold, try walking indoors at the gym or local mall or follow an exercise video on TV at home. (Always wear sunscreen, sunglasses, and a protective hat or visor on sunny days and, if it has rained recently, watch out for slippery surfaces.)

Wear the Right Athletic Shoe

A sturdy shoe is your best protection against injury during physical activity. Shoes don't have to be heavy to provide sufficient support, but

RICE for Exercise-Induced Injuries

If you don't treat an injury properly, you increase the chances that it will recur. To treat a minor muscle or ligament injury such as a sprained joint or strained muscle, use the RICE routine. RICE—which stands for rest, ice, compression, and elevation—will quickly relieve any pain and swelling. If the pain and swelling don't improve after using RICE for 48 hours, see your doctor. Don't exercise the affected area again until is has healed completely.

Rest

Resting an injured limb protects it from further injury and reduces the bleeding from damaged blood vessels, allowing the injury to heal. Avoid moving the injured area and don't put any weight on it for a while. Apply a sling to immobilize an injured shoulder or arm, and use crutches to shift weight off an injured leg or ankle.

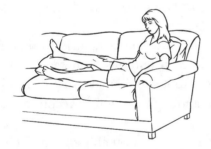

Ice

Place an ice pack on the injury as soon as you can. Apply ice for 20 minutes every hour you're awake for the first 24 to 48 hours after the injury. Cold helps relieve the pain and limit swelling and bruising by reducing both internal bleeding and the accumulation of fluid in the affected area.

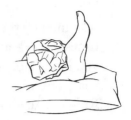

Compression

Compressing an injury helps to minimize swelling and speed healing. Wear an elastic bandage around the injured site for at least two days. You can wrap the bandage around an ice pack to apply cold to an injury and compress it at the same time. Wrap the bandage above and below the injury site evenly and tightly, but not too tightly; numbness, tingling, or increased pain at the site are signs that the bandage is too tight. Remove the compression bandage at night.

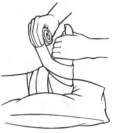

Elevation

Elevating an injured limb helps drain pooled fluid from the site and keeps bleeding and swelling to a minimum. Try to keep the injured area at a level higher than your heart. For example, elevate an injured leg with a pillow, especially at night, when your metabolism slows down. Place an injured arm in a sling.

thin-soled shoes such as canvas sneakers are probably not going to be sturdy enough to protect you from calf or Achilles-tendon problems. With the wide variety of athletic shoes available, you may be overwhelmed by the number of choices. If you walk or jog fewer than three times a week and infrequently play another sport, such as basketball, you'll probably be okay with an all-purpose cross-training shoe. Otherwise, buy a shoe that is designed for the activity you do most often. Runners need plenty of shock absorption, while walkers need footwear with extra cushioning at the heel. Basketball, racquetball, and tennis require shoes that provide ankle stability for twisting movements.

One important point to consider when choosing a shoe is whether your feet have high, medium, or low arches. If you have high arches, you tend to bear your weight on your heels and the balls of your feet. In this case, you should choose a cushioned shoe because it will absorb more of the shock when your foot hits the ground. People with low arches or flat feet need motion-control shoes because their feet move around inside their shoes, which could lead to an overuse injury. A medium arch requires both cushioning and motion control, so you should ask for a "stability" shoe. Your weight is a factor, too. If you weigh less than 150 pounds, you probably won't need as much stability in a shoe as a heavier person would.

The front part of the shoe, called the toe box, varies in height and width by style and brand. People with bunions, bone spurs, or other problems with the front part of the foot should make sure they select an athletic shoe that is wide enough and high enough to accommodate the problem.

Of course, the most important factor in buying an athletic shoe is proper fit. If you wear a shoe that does not fit properly, you will end up with blisters and calluses or, even worse, a sprained ankle or knee pain. If you have diabetes, foot sores and injuries can be a problem if your circulation has been affected. Here are some tips for getting properly fitting shoes:

- Have both feet measured, and pick the size that fits your larger foot. Most people's feet are not exactly the same size.
- Try on shoes at the end of the day, when your foot is at its widest.
- Wear your workout socks when trying on shoes.

- Make sure that you have a thumb's width of space between your longest toe and the end of the shoe's front.
- Check to see that your heels don't move up and down inside the shoe when you walk.

If you are very active, you should replace your athletic shoes every six months. Otherwise, get a new pair after you log about 300 miles on your shoes. Having trouble remembering exactly how long you've had those shoes? Write the date of purchase on the underside of the tongue of one of the shoes with permanent marker.

PART THREE

Diagnosing and Treating Type 2 Diabetes

6

How Do You Know If You Have Diabetes?

Many people are unaware that they have type 2 diabetes because they have no symptoms, especially in the early stages. Symptoms can also be so mild that they can go unnoticed for years. In fact, people have type 2 diabetes an average of four to seven years before it is detected. Experts believe that more than 5 million people in the United States have type 2 diabetes and don't know it.

You may have some of the symptoms of diabetes and think they are caused by something else. If you experience any of the warning signs of type 2 diabetes, no matter how mild, don't delay scheduling a checkup, even if you don't feel sick. You don't want to wait until you have severe complications such as nerve, kidney, or eye damage or heart problems before finding out you have diabetes. Generally, the earlier type 2 diabetes is diagnosed and treated, the more likely complications and tissue damage can be prevented or delayed.

Signs and Symptoms

Unlike type 1 diabetes, which comes on suddenly and produces obvious symptoms, type 2 diabetes usually develops without any noticeable symptoms, at least initially. Sometimes the symptoms develop gradually or appear to be harmless. For these reasons, type 2 diabetes can go undiagnosed for years. If you develop any of the following signs of type 2 diabetes, see your doctor right away. The earlier the condition is diagnosed and treatment begun, the less likely you are to develop major complications over the long term.

Intense Thirst

For most people, being thirsty is something that occurs when the weather is dry or excessively hot. For people who have untreated diabetes, thirst may be constant. They may wake up during the middle of the night to get a drink of water. Diabetes produces extreme thirst because the body is trying to compensate for the presence of a high level of sugar in the blood by sending a signal to the brain to water down the blood to dilute the sugar content and prevent dehydration. This mechanism translates into thirst that can't be quenched. Thirst is also a response to the excess water lost through increased urination, another common symptom of diabetes.

Increased Urination

One of the primary ways your body tries to cope with excess sugar in the blood is by eliminating it in urine. People with diabetes may have to urinate as often as once every hour and the symptom is especially noticeable and bothersome at night. The loss of so much water triggers more thirst, and the increased urination continues because of the high level of glucose in the blood. Fluid loss from excessive urination can lead to severe dehydration, a life-threatening condition in which the body does not have enough fluids for vital organs to function properly.

Extreme Hunger

People with diabetes often become extremely hungry and may lose weight even though they are eating normal amounts of food. The feelings of hunger result from the cells' not properly taking in glucose from food. Even though you are eating more, you don't gain weight and you may even lose weight because your body is not properly processing the calories you eat.

Fatigue

When your muscle cells don't have enough glucose to produce energy, you feel sluggish and tired. If you have already been diagnosed with type 2 diabetes, fatigue can be a red flag that tells you that your blood sugar is not under good control. Better management of your blood sugar may translate into less fatigue.

Unusual Weight Loss

People with diabetes may notice that they are losing weight without trying, even though they are consuming the same amount of food or more. Unexplained weight loss occurs because the body can't use glucose to produce energy, so it must resort to burning stored fat and protein. In addition, you may be losing several hundred calories a day of unused glucose in your urine. When stored fat gets used for fuel, you lose weight, but the weight loss includes an excessive loss of protein, a factor that contributes to the symptoms of weakness and fatigue.

Blurred Vision

An abrupt elevation in blood sugar levels can cause the lens of the eye to swell. This swelling can produce a sometimes sudden change in vision toward farsightedness. This means that a normally nearsighted person may actually see an improvement in distance vision without glasses, while a person who doesn't use glasses or who is already farsighted will see a blurring of his or her distance vision. Once blood sugar levels are under control, vision will return to normal within a few weeks.

Infections

High blood sugar can affect your immune system, making you more susceptible to infections, especially yeast infections of the genitals, skin infections, and urinary tract infections. High blood sugar also promotes the growth of bacteria. If you have diabetes and you are having frequent infections, your blood glucose may not be under good control. Check with your doctor about making adjustments in your treatment plan.

Sores That Don't Heal

People with diabetes often have circulation problems that cause poor blood flow to the legs and feet, reducing the delivery of oxygen and other nutrients to these tissues. High blood sugar also impairs the functioning of white blood cells, which defend against bacteria and are important for wound healing. Nerve problems can interfere with the sensation of pain so that minor skin irritations are not noticed or are ignored and can then worsen and become major problems. The elevated blood sugar levels that cause your body to lose fluids through urine can make your skin dry and cracked and susceptible to sores and bleeding. All of these factors can combine to produce sores that are slow to heal, especially on the feet.

Diagnostic Tests

To diagnose type 2 diabetes, doctors use blood tests to measure the level of glucose in the blood. Several factors, such as your level of activity and medications you are taking, can affect your blood sugar levels, so your doctor may perform more than one type of blood test before reaching a diagnosis. You will probably have some of the following tests if your doctor thinks you are at risk of developing type 2 diabetes or suspects you may already have it. Certain tests may need to be repeated to make sure the diagnosis is definite. It is also important to have regular blood tests to see if your cholesterol levels are within the normal range and to have your blood pressure taken frequently. Abnormal cholesterol levels and high blood pressure are major risk factors for heart disease and are especially common in people with type 2 diabetes.

Fasting Plasma Glucose Test

A fasting plasma glucose test measures your blood sugar level after you have fasted (have not had anything to eat or drink except water overnight or for at least 8 hours). The fasting plasma glucose test is a fairly reliable and convenient way to diagnose type 2 diabetes. It is most reliable when done in the morning. If your fasting blood sugar level is 100 to 125 milligrams per deciliter (mg/dL), you have a form of prediabetes (see page 14) called impaired fasting glucose. This means that, although you don't yet have type 2 diabetes, you are at high risk of developing it unless you make lifestyle changes. Levels over 125 mg/dL indicate a diagnosis of diabetes. The doctor will confirm the diagnosis by repeating the test. The chart below shows the diagnostic classifications from a fasting plasma glucose test based on blood glucose levels.

WHAT THE NUMBERS MEAN

Fasting Plasma Glucose Test Result	Diagnosis
60 to 99 mg/dL	Normal
100 to 125 mg/dL	Impaired fasting glucose (prediabetes)
126 mg/dL and above	Type 2 diabetes

Oral Glucose Tolerance Test

An oral glucose tolerance test measures your body's ability to use glucose. To prepare for the test, you may be asked to eat foods that are rich in carbohydrates (such as whole grains, cooked dried beans, and vegetables) for two or three days and then to fast overnight or for at least 8 hours.

The oral glucose tolerance test is more sensitive than the fasting plasma glucose test for diagnosing prediabetes and diabetes, but requires more effort. The amount of glucose in your blood plasma is measured just before you drink a liquid containing glucose dissolved in water and again 2 hours after drinking it. If your blood sugar level is between 140 and 190 mg/dL 2 hours after drinking the liquid, you have a form of prediabetes known as impaired glucose tolerance. This means that you don't yet have type 2 diabetes, but you are at high risk of developing it. A level of 200 mg/dL or above, confirmed by a repeat test, indicates that you have type 2 diabetes. This chart shows what the results of an oral glucose tolerance test indicate.

WHAT THE NUMBERS MEAN

Oral Glucose Tolerance Test Result	Diagnosis
139 mg/dL and below	Normal
140 to 199 mg/dL	Impaired glucose tolerance (prediabetes)
200 mg/dL and above	Type 2 diabetes

Doctors also use the oral glucose tolerance test to diagnose gestational diabetes, a form of diabetes that can develop in women during pregnancy. During pregnancy, your blood sugar levels will be checked four times during the glucose tolerance test. Levels that are above normal at least twice during the test confirm the diagnosis of gestational diabetes. For more about gestational diabetes, see chapter 15.

A1C Test

The hemoglobin A1C test, commonly called the A1C test, gives an indication of the average blood glucose level over the previous two to three months. This test provides information that lets your doctor understand how well your treatment plan is working over time. The test shows whether your blood sugar numbers have been close to normal or too high. The higher the level of glucose in your blood, the higher your A1C test result will be. High blood glucose levels increase your risk of serious health problems such as heart disease and nerve damage in the future.

Some of the glucose in your blood attaches to a protein called hemoglobin in your red blood cells, forming a substance called hemoglobin A1C. (Hemoglobin is the protein that carries oxygen from the lungs to all the tissues in the body.) The A1C test measures the percentage of this combined glucose-hemoglobin substance. Red blood cells live for three to four months. Once blood sugar combines with the hemoglobin in red blood cells, the A1C protein remains in the blood for the same amount of time and reveals how often blood sugar has risen and how high.

For example, if your blood sugar was high for a period of time several weeks ago, more glucose than usual combined with hemoglobin at that time. Even though your blood sugar levels may be closer to normal this week, your red blood cells retain the memory of the previous high blood sugar levels in the form of excess A1C.

You don't have to fast or prepare for the A1C test in any other way. At the doctor's office, your doctor or a lab technician will take a small blood sample and send it to a laboratory for testing. For most people with diabetes, an acceptable A1C result is less than 7. If your A1C number is less than 7, your treatment plan is probably working and your blood glucose is under control. If your A1C result is 8 or higher, your doctor will probably recommend some changes in your treatment plan to bring your A1C number down. Lowering your A1C number can improve your chances of staying healthy and reduce your risk of diabetic complications such as blindness, kidney disease, or nerve damage.

People with type 2 diabetes should have an A1C test at least twice a year. Your doctor may recommend having the test more often if you take insulin or if your blood glucose is not under good control. The A1C test is not meant to replace daily fingerstick testing with a glucose monitor. You still need to test your blood sugar as many times a day as your doctor recommends to make sure it stays at a healthy level.

Checking Your Blood Pressure

Blood pressure refers to the pressure exerted on the blood vessels as the heart pumps blood through the blood vessels. Blood pressure readings are taken using an instrument called a sphygmomanometer. A blood pressure reading is expressed in two numbers, which are usually written with a slash. For example, a blood pressure reading of 120/80 is usually stated as 120 over 80, a normal reading. The first number, or systolic blood pressure, is a measurement of the pressure in the blood vessels when the heart is beating. The second number, or diastolic blood pressure, is a measurement of the pressure in the vessels when the heart is at rest.

Blood pressure rises and falls throughout the day in response to stress, activity level, and many other factors. When it stays high all the time, it is diagnosed as high blood pressure, which doctors call hypertension. Nearly two out of three adults who have type 2 diabetes also have high blood pressure. Untreated diabetes and high blood pressure are an especially dangerous combination. On their own, high blood pressure and diabetes raise the risk of heart disease, stroke, eye disorders, kidney problems, and nerve damage. If you have both conditions, your risk of having these associated health problems is increased substantially if your blood pressure is not well controlled.

For this reason, if you have type 2 diabetes, make sure that your blood pressure is checked regularly (at least every six months), and if it is elevated, carefully follow the treatment your doctor recommends. Treating high blood pressure is essential for avoiding long-term complications. Even though high blood pressure does not cause symptoms in the early stages, it can damage blood vessels and other tissues throughout the body and increase your risk of heart attack and stroke.

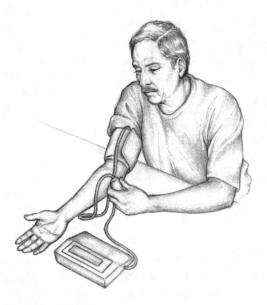

Measuring Blood Pressure

Your doctor may recommend that you purchase an automated blood pressure monitor to use regularly at home. Both mechanical and electronic blood pressure monitors are available at drugstores and through medical supply companies; ask your doctor which type you should buy. Bring your monitor with you to your doctor and ask the doctor or a nurse to show you how to use it correctly and to check it for accuracy. Some tips for getting reliable readings: always check your blood pressure at the same time every day, avoid caffeine and nicotine for at least 30 minutes before taking it, and relax in a quiet place for several minutes before taking it. If the reading is significantly higher or lower than the last one, wait a few minutes and take it again.

High blood pressure affects more than 65 million Americans and the risk increases with age; an estimated one out of two people over age 65 has high blood pressure. Yet as many as half of all people with high blood pressure do not know they have it because it does not cause symptoms early on.

Doctors usually advise people without diabetes whose blood pressure is slightly elevated and who have no additional risk factors for heart disease to make lifestyle changes in the areas of diet and exercise to try to bring their blood pressure down into the normal range. If these measures are not effective, doctors prescribe blood pressure medication. Most people who have diabetes and high blood pressure need to both make lifestyle changes and take medication to get their blood pressure below 120/80 and keep it there.

Most people with high blood pressure have what is referred to as essential hypertension. Essential hypertension has no known cause, but the following factors can increase your risk: having a family history of high blood pressure, being male or a woman past menopause, being overweight, being inactive, smoking cigarettes, being African American, drinking alcohol heavily, or experiencing severe or chronic stress. In some cases, high blood pressure can be caused by medical conditions such as kidney or thyroid disease or adrenal gland problems, or the use of illegal drugs such as cocaine.

Know Your Cholesterol Profile

Cholesterol is a fatty substance that is an essential component of cell membranes and is used by the body for insulating nerve fibers. Your body also needs a certain amount of cholesterol to make and transport fatty acids and to produce hormones and vitamin D. Problems arise when the amount of cholesterol in your blood gets too high, setting the stage for atherosclerosis (the buildup of fatty deposits in artery walls) and heart disease. Most of the cholesterol circulating in your blood is manufactured in your liver; the rest is absorbed from the fats in food you eat. You can control your cholesterol to some extent by limiting your intake of foods high in saturated and trans fats and cholesterol, which stimulate the liver to make more cholesterol. However, your cholesterol levels are largely influenced by genetic factors you inherited from your parents.

There are two major types of cholesterol in the blood: high-density lipoprotein (HDL) cholesterol, the so-called good cholesterol, and low-density lipoprotein (LDL) cholesterol , the bad cholesterol. High levels of LDL cholesterol cause fatty deposits to build up in the arteries, while HDL cholesterol helps clear the arteries of harmful LDL cholesterol. HDL and LDL levels need to be in a certain ratio to be beneficial: higher HDL levels and lower LDL levels are desirable. Many people with diabetes have cholesterol levels or ratios of LDL and HDL that are outside the healthy range—HDL levels that are too low or LDL levels that are too high, or both of these. These readings signal an increased risk of heart disease and stroke.

Beginning at age 20, you should have your cholesterol tested at least every five years—more frequently if you have a family history of heart disease or high cholesterol or if you have diabetes. Your cholesterol profile can help your doctor evaluate your risk of heart disease.

Often performed at the same time as a complete blood count (CBC) test, a cholesterol and lipids (blood fats) test evaluates the levels of different fats in your blood, including total cholesterol, HDL and LDL cholesterol, and triglycerides. Triglycerides are fats that store energy and are gradually released between meals to meet the body's requirements for fuel. Triglyceride testing is most reliable when performed after you have fasted for 12 hours.

Cholesterol and lipid levels can be affected by factors including obesity, menopause, diabetes, kidney or liver disease, hypothyroidism (an underactive thyroid gland), and drinking excessive amounts of alcohol. Some medications—including corticosteroids, diuretics ("water pills"), and birth-control pills—can also influence cholesterol numbers.

Total Cholesterol	Heart Disease Risk
Less than 200 mg/dL	Low risk
200–239 mg/dL	Borderline high risk
240 mg/dL and above	High risk

LDL (BAD) CHOLESTEROL

Less than 100 mg/dL	Low risk
100–129 mg/dL	Moderately low risk
130–159 mg/dL	Borderline high risk
160–189 mg/dL	High risk
190 mg/dL and above	Very high risk

HDL (GOOD) CHOLESTEROL

60 mg/dL and above	Low risk
50–59 mg/dL	Moderately low risk
40–49 mg/dL	Borderline high risk
39 mg/dL or less	High risk

TRIGLYCERIDES

Less than 150 mg/dL	Low risk
151–199 mg/dL	Borderline high risk
200–499 mg/dL	High risk
500 mg/dL and above	Very high risk

If your cholesterol profile is undesirable, your doctor will first prescribe a combination of healthful eating, increased physical activity, and weight loss to try to improve it. He or she will also encourage you to keep your blood sugar under control, which may help lower your LDL (bad) cholesterol and triglycerides.

If lifestyle measures are not effective in lowering your cholesterol to a healthy level, your doctor may prescribe a cholesterol-lowering medication. Several types of medications are available for controlling blood cholesterol. The most frequently prescribed cholesterol-lowering medications are the statins, which lower harmful LDL cholesterol, raise helpful HDL levels, and reduce high triglycerides by inhibiting an enzyme that controls the rate of cholesterol production by the liver.

7

Reaching a Healthy Weight

Reaching and maintaining a healthy weight is an essential goal for people with type 2 diabetes. Weight loss improves insulin sensitivity, enabling the insulin in your body to more easily lower blood sugar naturally. Losing weight will also help lower blood pressure and improve the levels of fats (lipids) circulating in the bloodstream, especially the harmful fats that can collect in artery walls and lead to a heart attack or a stroke.

Losing weight and keeping it off is undoubtedly one of the hardest things to do. Consider all the diet books at your local bookstore, each promising a quick, easy strategy for losing weight. But quick and easy is not the way to achieve safe and effective weight loss that you can maintain over the long term. The best way to lose weight is with the help and advice of your doctor and diabetes educator or dietitian, who can help you develop a meal plan that not only keeps your blood sugar levels near normal but also helps you lose weight and includes the foods you like to eat.

Midlife Weight Gain

During midlife, many people start to gain weight—or at least begin to find it harder to maintain their current weight. They also discover that the weight they gain is likely to accumulate around the abdominal area, which can make the body less sensitive to insulin and therefore less able to keep glucose at a healthy level. For women, these changes in weight usually begin during perimenopause (the years leading up to menopause), when levels of the female hormone estrogen start to decline. The average woman gains 1 pound each year during the years before menopause, but middle-age weight gain creeps up on men as well. The reasons for this shift in weight include the following factors:

- **Slower Metabolism** The chemical processes that enable your body to function begin to slow down in middle age, requiring less fuel. That means you need fewer calories from food than you did when you were younger. If you keep eating the same amount of calories without increasing your activity level, you will gain weight.

- **Lower Muscle Mass** As you age, your body composition shifts, giving you more fat and less muscle mass. Fat burns fewer calories than muscle, another reason you need fewer calories to maintain the same weight.

- **Less Physical Activity** Older people tend to exercise less than they did when they were younger, so they're burning fewer calories.

- **Inherited Factors** Genes have a strong influence on how much weight we gain as we age. But having a genetic tendency to put on weight does not mean that you are destined to gain weight as you age, provided you keep in mind that you need to reduce your calorie intake and increase your activity level. Inherited factors also affect how much weight we accumulate around the abdomen.

This excess weight can have harmful effects on your health, such as worsening your cholesterol profile, raising your blood pressure, making it harder to control your blood glucose, and increasing your risk of complications from diabetes.

How Weight Can Affect Diabetes

Carrying excess weight—especially around the abdomen—causes changes in the cells of the liver, body fat, and muscles, making them unable to use insulin properly. When cells are insensitive to the effects of insulin, they take in less glucose than normal and the level of glucose in the blood rises. In this situation, cells (such as cells in the eyes) that don't need insulin to take in glucose take in more than normal amounts of it. The excess glucose in these cells affects their ability to function and increases the likelihood of complications (such as the eye disease diabetic retinopathy; see page 183). Gradually, the liver also becomes unable to respond to insulin and starts to release more and more glucose into the bloodstream. Excess body fat and type 2 diabetes work hand in hand to create a cycle of increasing weight gain and decreasing sensitivity to insulin.

To treat your type 2 diabetes, your doctor will place you on a sensible weight-loss diet, such as a reduced-calorie version of the DASH diet (see page 119), which is prescribed for people with high blood pressure. Try to avoid fad diets, especially those that eliminate entire food groups, because they can be harmful to your health and might cause a deficiency in some essential nutrients.

In addition to the harmful effects that obesity can have on your diabetes and your general health, it can also negatively affect your quality of life. Your clothes don't fit, your self-esteem may suffer, and you may experience discrimination socially or in the workplace. Following are some of the ways in which being overweight can adversely affect your life. Let them help motivate you to work closely with your doctor, dietitian, or diabetes educator to start a weight-loss program now. In addition to improving your health, weight loss can significantly improve your quality of life as well as your self-esteem.

- **Ability to Function**   Severely obese adults and children may not be able to run or walk very far without getting out of breath. As a result, they become less active, which in turn makes them likely to put on more weight. Being overweight also puts excess stress on the joints, which, over time, can lead to osteoarthritis. Osteoarthritis can be painful and may affect mobility. These limitations can have an influence on a person's independence and quality of life.

- **Employment**   People who are overweight—especially women—are disproportionately subject to discrimination at every stage of employment, including hiring, compensation, promotion, discipline, and termination.

- **Self-image**   Being overweight can hinder social interactions and relationships, causing anxiety, loneliness, and, in some cases, depression.

- **Financial Consequences**   Not only do you earn less on average when you are overweight, you may also have to pay more for items such as health insurance and life insurance, and you may need to purchase adaptive devices to help you perform your daily activities.

Weight-Loss Strategies

Doctors consider weight loss to be successful if it results in at least a 10-percent reduction in weight that is maintained for at least one year. There are hundreds of fad diets, and people continue to try extreme measures, but only a few sensible strategies have been proven to be successful. Always keep in mind that the bottom line for weight loss is one simple formula: eat less and exercise more over the long term. Aside from eating less and exercising more, the weight-loss options most often recommended for permanent weight loss are behavior therapy, medication, modified fasting, and weight-loss surgery.

Behavior Therapy

Psychiatrists and psychologists use behavior therapy to change the negative belief patterns and behaviors of the overweight people they treat. The method has been as successful for helping with weight loss as it has been for treating psychiatric disorders such as anxiety and depression. The cornerstone of behavior therapy for weight loss is a strategy known as self-monitoring—the systematic observation and recording of eating and exercise activities. For example, your doctor may recommend that you reduce your fat intake to a certain number of grams per day. To do this, you would need to read food labels to determine how much fat you consume in each serving of food and write the amounts down in a food diary. You might also have to engage in a certain amount of exercise every day, say 10,000 steps. To reach this exercise goal, your doctor will probably recommend that you use a pedometer, a small mechanical device that attaches to a waistband or a belt and measures and records the number of steps you take.

In addition to tracking your eating and exercise patterns every day, behavior therapy teaches you to do the following:

- Recognize high-risk situations (such as having favorite high-calorie snacks in the house) and avoid them.

- Reward yourself for exercising longer than expected or eating less of a certain food or less at a meal.
- Alter false beliefs about your body image.
- Round up a support network of family members and friends.
- Join an organized support group where you can meet people who motivate one another to reach their weight-loss goals and maintain them over the long term.

Another powerful behavior-changing tactic is the use of mindfulness exercises to raise the awareness of your body's hunger and fullness cues. We often eat without thinking about it, especially when we're faced with a favorite sweet or snack or a table full of high-fat, high-calorie appetizers. It's also easy to overeat when we're doing something else, such as watching TV, at the same time and not focusing on eating. Many overweight people frequently eat when they aren't hungry and continue eating after they are full because they tend to use food as a way to meet their emotional needs.

Mindfulness exercises can help you keep focused "in the moment" as you eat, allowing you to taste your food fully and concentrate on the sensations that are occurring inside your body from moment to moment, rather than on your emotional state. These exercises have been shown to reduce binge-eating and increase self-control while eating. Your doctor may also recommend daily meditation (see page 129) to relieve stress and put you in a comfortable state of nonjudgmental awareness in which you can become even more in tune with what is happening inside your body.

For people for whom behavior therapy alone is not effective in promoting weight loss, doctors may prescribe appetite-suppressing medications, antidepressants, supervised fasting, or even surgery to boost its effectiveness.

Weight-Loss Medications

Your doctor may consider weight-loss medication if your body mass index (BMI, see page 35) is higher than 30, but he or she will be cautious in prescribing medication because some weight-loss medications used in the past have produced serious side effects. Don't harbor any illusions that a weight-loss medication will miraculously melt those pounds away. You will still have to cut back on calories, consume a healthy diet, and be more physically active. Keep in mind that none of these medications has been approved for lifelong use; they are prescribed for only a limited amount of time specified by your doctor. Researchers are working on developing weight-loss and weight-maintenance medications that can be used for life, just as lifelong therapy is needed to control hypertension, diabetes, and high cholesterol.

Many weight-loss medications are used in combination with behavior therapy (see page 100) to make the therapy even more effective. Following are the medications that are most commonly prescribed for weight loss:

- **Orlistat** This medication works by inhibiting the body's absorption of fat from food.
- **Phentermine** This appetite suppressant was one of the two ingredients in the problematic weight-loss drug combination fen-phen, which was taken off the market because of safety concerns. However, the use of phentermine alone does not seem to produce the adverse effects on the heart that fen-phen did.
- **Sibutramine** Doctors prescribe this medication for appetite suppression.

Make sure you see your doctor on a regular basis while taking any weight-loss medication so he or she can monitor how well it is working and make sure you aren't experiencing any harmful side effects.

Very Low Calorie Diet

A very low calorie diet is an approach that combines severe calorie restriction with protein intake to produce rapid weight loss in severely obese people. A form of the diet using liquid protein was popular in the late 1970s but quickly lost favor after being blamed for a series of unexplained sudden deaths. Apparently the contents of the liquid protein used at that time was of poor quality and supplied mainly by gelatin, and the products were too readily available over the counter. Today the approach is used exclusively under a doctor's strict supervision and the liquid protein products are sold only to doctors and hospitals. Modified fasting is recommended solely for people who are dangerously overweight.

If your doctor places you on a very low calorie diet, he or she will prescribe a daily intake of 75 to 100 grams of protein, either in the form of meat or liquid protein, while restricting total calorie intake to about

600 calories a day. The process can produce a number of side effects, including:

- Fatigue
- Light-headedness
- Constipation
- Dry skin
- Intolerance of cold
- Irregular heartbeat
- Potassium deficiency
- Hair loss

A very low calorie diet is considered a strict and disciplined regimen that requires careful monitoring through frequent medical checkups and behavior therapy (see page 100). If your doctor places you on this regimen, be sure to keep all of your follow-up appointments so he or she can evaluate your health and monitor the effectiveness of the weight-loss program. Report any side effects—especially heartbeat irregularities—to your doctor right away.

Weight-Loss Surgery

Weight-loss surgery, also known as bariatric surgery or gastrointestinal surgery for obesity, is targeted to people with extreme obesity—a body mass index (BMI; see page 35) of at least 40, or about 80 pounds over-weight for most women and 100 pounds overweight for most men. People who have a BMI between 35 and 39.9 and a serious obesity-related health problem—such as type 2 diabetes, heart disease, or sleep apnea (the periodic cessation of breathing during sleep)—may also be candidates for weight-loss surgery. As with any weight-loss strategy, success in maintaining weight loss over the long term requires lifestyle changes including eating healthfully and engaging in regular physical activity.

Doctors have developed three main weight-loss surgical approaches: restrictive surgery (which limits food intake), malabsorptive surgery (which blocks the absorption of nutrients by the intestines), and a combination of these two. The combination procedures are performed most frequently and have the best weight-loss success rate. Malabsorptive surgery alone is no longer recommended because it can cause severe nutritional deficiencies.

Restrictive surgery limits food intake by creating a narrow passage from the upper part of the stomach into the lower part, reducing the amount of food the stomach can hold and slowing the passage of food through the stomach. To perform this operation, surgeons use a silicone band to create a small pouch at the top of the stomach, where food enters from the esophagus. This band—about a half inch in diameter— slows the rate at which food empties from the pouch into the lower part of the stomach. It also produces a feeling of fullness soon after swallowing, which helps prevent a person from eating large amounts of food at one time. Food has to be soft, moist, and well-chewed before it is swallowed, which significantly slows the eating process (another way to reduce food intake).

Restrictive surgery can be done laparoscopically, using small abdominal incisions through which the surgical instruments are passed. One of the most common side effects of restrictive weight-loss surgery is vomiting after eating too much. The restrictive band can also slip out of place or wear away, requiring additional surgery. People typically lose 50 to 60 percent of their excess weight, but many people gain back much of the weight within 10 years if they haven't adopted a lifetime plan of healthy eating and regular physical activity.

Malabsorptive surgery does not inhibit food intake. Instead, digested food bypasses most of the small intestine, where absorption of nutrients takes place, reducing the amount of nutrients and calories that are absorbed. No longer recommended to be used alone (because of the risk of nutritional deficiencies), malabsorptive surgery is combined with restrictive surgery in a procedure called gastric bypass.

In one gastric bypass procedure, the surgeon creates a small stomach pouch to restrict food intake (restrictive surgery) and then attaches a Y-shaped section of the small intestine to the pouch so food can bypass the lower stomach and the first and second segments of the small intestine, reducing the amount of nutrients and calories the body can absorb.

Most people who have the combined surgery lose weight quickly and keep losing weight for up to two years. Because the combined surgery produces greater weight loss than restrictive surgery alone, it is more likely to improve the health problems that accompany obesity, such as glucose intolerance and type 2 diabetes, heart disease, high blood pressure, abnormal blood fats, and sleep apnea.

Weight-loss surgery is not without risks and potential complications. The combined procedures are riskier than the restrictive procedures and are more likely to cause long-term nutritional deficiencies. Almost 1 in 20 patients has serious cardiovascular problems after gastric bypass surgery, including heart attack, stroke, or severe high blood pressure, and 1 in 200 dies within 30 days of having the procedure. Cost for the procedures can range from $20,000 to $50,000; health insurance coverage varies by state and insurance provider.

8

Eating a Healthy Diet

Healthful eating is a cornerstone of diabetes management. In fact, it is so important that your doctor will probably refer you to a registered dietitian (a health professional who is an expert in diet and nutrition) or a diabetes educator (a health professional who is certified to teach people with diabetes how to manage it). The dietitian or diabetes educator will develop a meal plan adapted to your specific needs that also takes into consideration your lifestyle and the kinds of foods you like to eat. He or she will probably also consider your ethnic and cultural background when developing your meal plan.

One of the most important things you will learn is when and how to eat the right kinds of carbohydrates, because carbohydrates have the biggest effect on blood sugar levels. Your meal plan will also focus on controlling calories to help you lose weight if you are overweight. For many people with type 2 diabetes, weight loss and increased physical activity are the most effective ways to bring their glucose down to a healthy level and keep it there.

Your Meal Plan

When you have type 2 diabetes, the type and amount of food you eat and when you eat each affects your blood sugar levels. Blood sugar levels go up after eating. You should try to eat about the same amount of food at about the same time each day to keep your blood glucose near normal levels. If you eat a big dinner one day and a small dinner the next, your blood glucose levels may fluctuate too much. The following general eating guidelines can help you keep your blood glucose at a healthy level:

- Eat about the same amount of food every day.
- Consume your meals and snacks at about the same times each day.
- Don't skip meals (or snacks if they have been recommended).
- If you take diabetes medication, take it at the same time every day.
- Exercise the same amount at about the same time each day.

There is no single diet that is right for everyone. Your doctor and dietitian or diabetes educator will develop a meal plan that is right for you. Consistent timing of your meals and snacks may not be as important as it is for someone with type 1 diabetes who is taking insulin, but keeping blood sugar levels near normal is just as important.

Carbohydrates (see page 47) are especially important because they have the biggest influence on blood glucose. Eat about the same amount of carbohydrate-rich foods at about the same time each day. Starches (such as whole-grain bread, cereal, rice, and pasta), fruits, milk, and starchy vegetables such as corn and potatoes are all good sources of carbohydrates. Make sure your starches come from whole grains because they contain fiber and many other nutrients and are digested and absorbed by the body more slowly than refined starches, helping to keep blood glucose steady.

While carbohydrates are an important focus of your meal plan, protein and healthy fats are also important. Your dietitian or diabetes educator will carefully calculate the correct ratio of these nutrients. The typical recommendations are 45 to 65 percent of total calories from carbohydrates, 12 to 20 percent from protein, and less than 30 percent from fat (including healthy fats). Depending on your circumstances, your doctor may recommend slightly different percentages for you.

How much of each type of food you need depends on how many calories you need each day to lose weight or maintain a healthy weight (see page 37). Avoid high-fat foods and sweets because they provide a lot of calories but few nutrients. To make sure your food servings are the right size, use measuring cups and spoons and a food scale. Keeping track of your calorie intake can help you keep your blood sugar at a steady level and can help you make adjustments for reaching weight goals.

To develop a meal plan that fits your needs, your dietitian or diabetes educator will ask you questions about your lifestyle and your personal food preferences. He or she can help you plan meals that include foods that are not only good for you but that are also familiar foods that you and your family like to eat. The biggest dangers for people with type 2 diabetes are cardiovascular (heart and blood vessel) problems, which can lead to heart attack or stroke. Circulation problems also cause poor blood flow to the legs and feet. To prevent these problems, your dietitian or diabetes educator will teach you about heart-healthy eating that can help you reduce your risk for or avoid heart and blood vessel disease. Your meal plan will probably include the following recommendations:

- Eat foods that are low in saturated fat and have no trans fats; no more than 7 to 10 percent of your total daily calorie intake should come from saturated fat. Buy prepared foods with less than 1 gram of saturated fat per serving.

- Limit your intake of foods that are high in cholesterol, such as egg yolks. Consume no more than 300 milligrams of cholesterol a day, or 200 milligrams if you have heart disease.

- Don't eat too much salt; buy reduced-sodium or "no salt added" prepared foods. Look for prepared foods with less than 140 milligrams of sodium per serving or 5 percent of the "daily value" for sodium on the food label.

- Consume 9 to 13 servings of fruits and vegetables each day; whole fruits and vegetables are more nutritious and less calorie-dense than juices and dried fruit.

- Boost your fiber intake by eating whole grains, dried beans (legumes), fruits, and vegetables.

- Limit added sugars to less than 25 percent of your total daily calories. These sugars, which are added to foods (such as pastries, candy, and other sweets) and beverages (such as soft drinks and fruit drinks) during production, usually provide few nutrients but lots of calories.

Carbohydrates Are Key

The goal of your meal plan is to keep your blood sugar level as close to normal as possible after and between meals. It is important to be aware of how much carbohydrate you are eating, because carbohydrates have the greatest effect on blood sugar levels. Careful carbohydrate planning to keep blood sugar balanced, combined with eating foods that are low in total, saturated, and trans fats, can help lower your heart disease risk and your risk of complications from diabetes.

Carbohydrates are supplied primarily by grains, starchy foods such corn and potatoes, fruit, and milk. Vegetables also have some carbohydrate content, but protein foods, oils, and fats contain very little carbohydrate. Always try to consume carbohydrates that are high in fiber because they are digested slowly and therefore tend to keep blood sugar levels more stable.

How much carbohydrate should you eat? The amount needed varies from person to person. Also important is the distribution of your carbohydrate intake throughout the day in both meals and snacks. Your doctor, dietitian, or diabetes educator will decide how much carbohydrate you should have at each meal or snack depending on your weight and height, activity level, age, and any medications you are taking. The results of tests for blood sugar and cholesterol and triglycerides will also influence your daily carbohydrate count recommendation.

To keep good control of your blood sugar levels, you will have to learn how to be consistent in the type, amount, and timing of the carbohydrates you eat throughout the day and from day to day. The two methods that people with diabetes use to keep track of their daily intake of carbohydrates and other nutrients are dietary exchanges and carbohydrate counting (see page 114).

Fiber and Blood Sugar Control

You should definitely consume a lot more high-fiber foods. Fiber (see page 47) is especially beneficial for people with type 2 diabetes because it can help keep blood glucose levels steady. There are two types of fiber in the food you eat: water soluble and water insoluble. Neither type of fiber is digestible, but they both play an important role in your diet. Of the two types, soluble fiber has the strongest effect on blood sugar. Foods rich in soluble fiber are digested gradually, slowing down the absorption of glucose into the blood. The result is smaller increases in blood sugar after eating.

Soluble fiber has another possible health benefit: reducing your risk of heart disease. It lowers total blood cholesterol as well as harmful LDL cholesterol by absorbing cholesterol from the bloodstream and excreting it as waste. Soluble fiber may also reduce the amount of cholesterol your liver produces.

Foods that contain high amounts of soluble fiber include grains such as oat bran, oatmeal, barley, and rye; fruits such as blackberries, oranges, apples, and pears; beans and legumes (including kidney beans, black-eyed peas, lentils, split peas, and soybeans); flaxseed; and psyllium (a grass found in some cereal products and breads, some dietary supplements, and some over-the-counter stool softeners and laxatives).

Doctors recommend that most people—including those without diabetes—get 20 to 40 grams of fiber every day. Up to age 50, the recommendation is up to 40 grams a day for men and 25 grams a day for women. After age 50, men are advised to consume 30 grams and women 20 grams daily (because people usually eat less as they get older). Children should have a daily fiber intake equal to their age plus 5 grams per day; for example, an 8-year-old child should eat 8 plus 5 grams, or 13 grams.

These figures may seem daunting, but you'll find that it's not so difficult if you add fiber to your diet gradually. Start by buying some high-fiber breakfast cereals that contain whole grains or flaxseed. Prepare more fiber-rich dishes such as bean soups, stews, and casseroles. Toss some chickpeas or other beans into your salads. For a side dish, serve black-eyed peas instead of a starch such as potatoes or rice. And, of course, eat lots of fruits and vegetables.

The same foods that contain soluble fiber also supply insoluble fiber in varying amounts. Insoluble fiber increases stool bulk, speeds up the time it takes stool to travel through the intestines, and improves bowel regularity. At the same time, fiber may also reduce your risk of colon cancer, hemorrhoids, and digestive disorders.

You should be aware, however, that dietary fiber can influence the effect of some common medications. For example, a high fiber intake can lower the body's absorption of cholesterol-reducing medications called HMG-CoA reductase inhibitors, the heart medication digoxin, and lithium (prescribed for bipolar disorder). If you take any of these prescription medications, talk to your doctor before increasing your fiber intake.

Dietary Exchanges

The dietary exchange system was developed by the American Diabetes Association and the American Dietetic Association to help people with diabetes plan their meals to gain better control over their blood glucose levels. The system divides food into three main groups: carbohydrates, meat and meat substitutes, and fats. Each group contains a subgroup of foods that are similar in calorie, carbohydrate, protein, and fat content to make the same foods in a list virtually interchangeable. For example, under carbohydrates, you'll find that one fruit exchange supplies 15 grams of carbohydrates and about 60 calories. Fruits corresponding to one fruit exchange include 1 cup of blueberries, 1 small apple, or 1 medium peach. Under the meat exchanges category, one very lean meat exchange equals 7 grams of protein, 0 to 3 grams of fat, and 35 calories. For the very lean meat exchange, you can choose 1 ounce of chicken or turkey white meat with no skin, ¼ cup of low-fat cottage cheese, or 2 egg whites.

A dietitian or diabetes educator develops a meal plan that contains a certain number of exchanges for each day depending on a person's weight, height, age, medical history, and whether weight loss is part of the plan. Forty-five to 65 percent of total calorie intake each day should come from carbohydrates, your body's main source of fuel.

Following is a chart showing the dietary exchanges that you can use to help you follow your meal plan and manage your diabetes. As you can see, choosing fat-free milk or very lean poultry instead of whole-fat milk and beef or pork cuts a lot of calories that you can save up for another meal or apply toward your weight-loss plan.

FIGURING EXCHANGES

Exchange	Nutrient Content	Equivalent Foods
CARBOHYDRATE EXCHANGES		
One starch	15 grams carbohydrate 3 grams protein 1 gram (or less) fat	1 slice bread; ¼ bagel; ¾ cup cold cereal; ⅓ cup rice, pasta, or cooked dried beans; 3-ounce potato
One fruit exchange	15 grams carbohydrate 60 calories	1 small apple, banana, or orange; 1 medium peach; 1 cup fresh berries; 4 ounces unsweetened juice
One fat-free or low-fat milk exchange	12 grams carbohydrate 8 grams protein 0–3 grams fat 90 calories	1 cup fat-free milk; ¾ cup plain fat-free or low-fat yogurt

Exchange	Nutrient Content	Equivalent Foods
CARBOHYDRATE EXCHANGES		
One reduced-fat milk exchange	12 grams carbohydrate 8 grams protein 5 grams fat 120 calories	1 cup 2% milk; 1 cup soy milk
One whole-milk exchange	12 grams carbohydrates 8 grams protein 8 grams fat 150 calories	1 cup whole milk; $3/4$ cup plain whole-milk yogurt
One nonstarchy vegetable exchange	5 grams carbohydrate 2 grams protein 0 gram fat 25 calories	$1/2$ cup cooked vegetables; 1 cup raw vegetables or salad greens; $1/2$ cup vegetable juice
Other carbohydrate exchange	15 grams carbohydrate, with varying amounts of protein, fat, and calories	1 tablespoon jelly or table sugar; a dessert such as $1/2$ cup frozen yogurt
MEAT AND MEAT SUBSTITUTE EXCHANGES		
One very lean protein exchange	7 grams protein 0–1 gram fat 35 calories	1 ounce poultry white meat; tuna canned in water; 2 egg whites; $3/4$ cup low-fat cottage cheese
One lean protein exchange (limit to twice a week)	7 grams protein 3 grams fat 55 calories	1 ounce poultry dark meat; lean beef, pork, or lamb; low-fat cheese
One medium-fat protein exchange (choose very infrequently)	7 grams protein 5 grams fat 75 calories	1 ounce beef or pork; 1 whole egg; 1 ounce mozzarella cheese
One high-fat protein exchange (ask your doctor how often you can eat these)	7 grams protein 8 grams fat 100 calories	1 ounce whole-fat cheese; 1 ounce spare ribs; 1 tablespoon peanut butter
FAT EXCHANGES		
One fat exchange	5 grams fat 45 calories	1 teaspoon oil or butter; 1 tablespoon salad dressing or cream cheese; $1/8$ avocado
FREE EXCHANGES		
One free food exchange	Less than or equal to 5 grams carbohydrate or less than 20 calories	Many vegetables, including celery, lettuce, spinach, cabbage, cucumbers, and zucchini, when eaten in moderation (1 to 2 servings per meal); most condiments, such as 1 table-spoon ketchup; desserts such as sugar-free gelatin

Carbohydrate Counting

An alternative to the food exchanges method for managing food intake to regulate blood sugar is known as carbohydrate counting, which computes the grams of carbohydrates you consume throughout the day. The logic behind carb counting is that all carbohydrates—whether they're nutritious foods such as whole grains and fruit or non-nutritious foods such as sugary soft drinks and candy—have a similar effect on blood sugar levels. For this reason, the total amount of carbohydrates is the most important factor, not the particular food.

With carb counting, you don't have to figure out how each food corresponds to the traditional exchange meal plan; you just need to know how much carbohydrate it contains. Purchase a good pocket reference book or pamphlet that shows how many carbohydrates are in a serving of fresh or unpackaged foods such as produce. Using a food scale and measuring cups and spoons to measure food servings can help you learn to eyeball serving sizes (see page 119). Counting carbohydrates can help make your carbohydrate intake more precise, leading to greater control of your blood glucose.

Counting the grams of carbohydrates you need each day makes it easy to plan meals because all you have to do is look at the nutrition label on a packaged food or the nutrient analysis box on a recipe to see how many grams of carbohydrates it contains. (Watch serving sizes so you don't inadvertently consume more than one serving and miscalculate your carb count.)

To simplify the task even more, many people count the carbohydrate content of one serving of starch, fruit, or milk as 15 grams. Three servings of nonstarchy vegetables are also counted as 15 grams, and you don't need to count one or two servings of nonstarchy vegetables— they're considered free carbs. Each meal or snack should supply a certain number of carbohydrate grams, according to your meal plan. Let's say your meal-plan breakfast is supposed to have four servings of carbohydrates, which translates into 60 total grams of carbohydrates for that meal. Looking at your box of shredded wheat, you see that one serving contains 30 grams of carbohydrates (make sure you don't exceed one serving). One cup of milk adds another 15 grams, bringing your carb count to 45 grams. A small apple or pear adds another 15 grams, for a total of 60 grams. If you also eat a 2-ounce serving of cheese at breakfast, it will not add to your carbohydrate count because cheese contains little carbohydrate.

Glycemic Index

Another school of thought says that all carbohydrates are not created equal and that some that break down quickly in the intestine raise blood sugar too fast. This ranking of carbohydrates is called the glycemic index, a system that rates carbohydrate foods by their effects on blood sugar. Carbohydrates that break down rapidly in the bloodstream have a high glycemic index; those that break down more slowly have a lower glycemic index. Eating lower-glycemic-index foods can result in a smaller rise in blood sugar after meals, the theory goes.

The following are examples of foods that are high on the glycemic index and, therefore, are thought to raise blood sugar levels quickly:

- White rice
- White bread
- White potatoes
- Saltine crackers
- Orange juice
- Pastas made from white flour

Examples of low-glycemic-index foods include:

- Whole-grain breads and cereals
- Oatmeal (not instant)
- Sweet potatoes
- Cooked dried beans, peas, and lentils
- Fresh fruit

Many doctors don't consider the glycemic index an essential tool for helping people regulate their blood sugar because the body's response to eating is much more complicated than the glycemic index suggests. For example, different people digest food at different rates, so a given food can make one person's blood sugar level go up faster than that of another person. Also, your body's blood sugar response to eating a food depends on such factors as the type of food, how much you consumed, how it was cooked or processed, and whether you ate fat or protein with it. Age and activity level also influence how a certain food can affect blood sugar.

Dietary Guidelines for Americans

Much chronic illness in the United States, including type 2 diabetes, is linked to a poor diet and a sedentary lifestyle. The Dietary Guidelines for Americans, published jointly by the US Department of Health and Human Services and the US Department of Agriculture, are designed to provide common-sense recommendations to promote good health and reduce the risk of disease through a balanced, varied diet and regular physical activity.

A basic premise of the Dietary Guidelines is that nutrients should be consumed primarily through food. Healthful foods contain a variety of nutrients that have beneficial effects on health. Fortified foods and dietary supplements may be useful in providing nutrients that might otherwise be consumed in insufficient amounts, but dietary supplements can never replace a healthy diet. The Dietary Guidelines advise taking action to improve your health by following these nine recommendations:

1. **Get adequate nutrients within your calorie needs.** Choose a variety of high-nutrient foods and beverages. Limit your intake of foods containing saturated and trans fats, cholesterol, added sugar, salt, and alcohol.

2. **Manage your weight.** To keep your weight within a healthy range, don't regularly consume more calories than you expend each day. To prevent gradual weight gain as you age, increase your level of physical activity.

3. **Get 30 to 90 minutes of physical activity each day.** Perform 30 minutes of exercise to 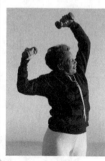 lower your risk of chronic disease, 60 minutes to prevent weight gain in adulthood, and 90 minutes to lose weight. Include aerobic exercise to strengthen your heart, stretching exercises to increase flexibility, and resistance exercises for muscle strength.

4. **Boost your intake of certain food groups.** Each day, consume the equivalent of 2 cups of fruit and 2½ cups of vegetables for a 2,000-calorie diet. Include plant foods from the dark green, orange, starch, and legume groups each week. At least half of your grain foods should come from whole grains. Consume 3 cups of fat-free or low-fat milk or other dairy products a day.

5. **Know your fats.**
   - Maintain your saturated fat intake below 10 percent of total calories, and consume less than 300 mg of cholesterol each day. Keep trans fat consumption as low as possible.
   - Your total fat intake should range between 20 and 35 percent of calories, with most fats coming from the polyunsaturated and monounsaturated varieties.
   - Select lean meats and poultry and fat-free dairy products.

6. **Be smart about carbohydrates.** Boost your intake of fiber from whole grains, fruits, and vegetables. Don't add sugar to foods and beverages. Consume sugar-containing foods and beverages infrequently.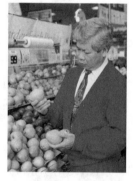

7. **Restrict sodium intake and get sufficient potassium.** Limit your intake of salt to 1 teaspoon (2,300 mg) per day; 1,500 mg if you are middle aged or older, have high blood pressure, or are African American. Increase your consumption of potassium-rich fruits and vegetables (such as bananas, oranges, greens, peas, and tomatoes).

8. **Drink alcohol in moderation, if at all.** Limit alcohol consumption to two drinks a day for

men and one drink a day for women. Don't drink alcohol at all if you are alcoholic, pregnant, trying to become pregnant, breast-feeding, or a minor, or if you take medications that can interact with alcohol or you have certain medical conditions, such as liver disease.

9. Prepare and store food safely.

- Wash your hands before and after preparing food. Wash all fruits and vegetables before preparing.
- Keep raw foods separate from other foods while shopping for, preparing, or storing them.
- Cook food thoroughly to kill dangerous microorganisms.
- Avoid unpasteurized milk and juices; raw eggs; undercooked meat, poultry, fish, and shellfish; and raw sprouts.

Special Recommendations for Older Adults

Because older adults tend to eat less than younger people, many do not get sufficient amounts of some key vitamins, especially vitamin D (which maintains bone strength) and vitamin B12 (which maintains nerve function and oxygen-carrying red blood cells). Some signs of vitamin B12 deficiency include fatigue, weakness, loss of appetite, and weight loss, and neurological changes such as numbness and tingling in the hands and feet, difficulty maintaining balance, depression, confusion, dementia, and poor memory. To prevent these problems and maintain bone strength, which tends to decrease with age, the FDA recommends that older people do the following:

- Consume extra vitamin D from fortified foods (such as milk) or supplements.
- Get enough vitamin B12 from fortified foods (such as breakfast cereals) or supplements.
- Get regular exercise to reduce the decline in function that can come with age.

Special Recommendations for Pregnant Women

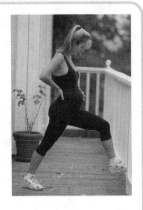

Pregnancy puts extra nutritional demands on a woman because her body is providing nutrients for the developing fetus. The following recommendations can help you stay healthy during your pregnancy and help ensure that your baby is born healthy:

- Consume enough folic acid (a B vitamin) to prevent birth defects.
- Get 30 minutes of moderate physical activity but avoid activities with a high risk for falls or abdominal injury.
- Make sure you gain enough weight, as recommended by your doctor.

Special Recommendations for Children

Because lifestyle factors contribute to common chronic disorders, including type 2 diabetes and heart disease, the FDA is recommending that parents help children adopt healthy habits with the following recommendations. The focus is on helping children avoid becoming overweight, the most important step in preventing type 2 diabetes.

- Get at least 1 hour of physical activity every day.
- Avoid weight-loss diets (unless recommended by a doctor). Instead, increase physical activity and limit high-calorie foods.
- Don't limit fat consumption until 2 years of age. Keep fat consumption between 30 and 35 percent for children between ages 2 and 3.
- Give children ages 2 to 8 two cups per day of fat-free milk or dairy products; children over the age of 9 years should consume 3 cups.

Because carbohydrates, both simple and complex, have the biggest influence on blood sugar levels, it is important to keep track of the grams of carbohydrates you eat each day. But the type of carbohydrate you eat matters for a different reason. You should try to eat primarily nutrient-dense ("low-glycemic") carbohydrates such as whole grains, fruits, vegetables, and fat-free dairy products. Limit refined and processed ("high-glycemic") carbohydrate-containing foods such as white bread, white rice, pasta made with white flour, and cookies and other sweets primarily because they pack a lot of calories but provide few other nutrients.

How Many Calories Do You Need?

It may be hard to figure out exactly how much you need to eat each day to maintain a healthy weight or to lose weight. The number of calories you need each day depends on your gender, your body frame, how much you weigh, and how physically active you are. Your doctor, dietitian, or diabetes educator will tell you how many calories you need to consume each day, but as a general rule the following guidelines can be helpful.

FIGURING YOUR CALORIES

If you are	Your total daily calories should be	You should consume the following
A small woman who exercises or a small to medium-sized woman who wants to lose weight or a medium-sized woman who doesn't exercise much	1,200 to 1,600	6 starches 3 vegetables 2 fruits 2 milk or yogurt servings 2 meat or fish servings up to 3 healthy fats
A large woman who wants to lose weight or a small man of normal weight or a medium-sized man who leads a sedentary life or a medium-sized to large man who wants to lose weight	1,600 to 2,000	8 starches 4 vegetables 3 fruits 2 milk or yogurt servings 2 meat or fish servings up to 4 healthy fats
A medium-sized to large man who exercises a lot or has a physically active job such as construction work or a large man of normal weight or a large woman who exercises a lot or has a physically demanding job	2,000 to 2,400	11 starches 4 vegetables 3 fruits 2 milk or yogurt servings 2 meat or fish servings up to 5 healthy fats

Controlling Portion Sizes

Weighing and measuring foods with a food scale, measuring cups, and measuring spoons will help you eat just the right amount at each meal. The following tips can teach you how to eyeball serving sizes once you become familiar with a typical meal-plan serving:

- Measure a serving of cooked pasta or rice or dry cereal into a bowl or plate. The next time you eat the same food, use the same bowl or plate and fill it to the same level.
- Measure one serving of milk into a glass and see how high it fills the glass. Always drink milk out of the same size glass, filled to the same level.
- One 3-ounce serving of meat or other protein is about the size of a deck of cards.
- One ounce of meat or cheese is equivalent to the size of your thumb.
- One teaspoon is about the size of the tip of your thumb.
- One serving of starch is 1 slice of bread, 1 small potato, ½ cup cooked breakfast cereal or ¾ cup dry cereal, or 1 small (6-inch) tortilla.

The DASH Eating Plan

Developed by scientists from the National Heart, Lung, and Blood Institute, the Dietary Approaches to Stop Hypertension (DASH) eating plan is a sensible and proven way to lower blood pressure. Yes, you can actually reduce your blood pressure by following this diet, which is low in total fat, saturated fat, trans fats, and cholesterol; low in salt; and rich in fruits, vegetables, and fat-free dairy products.

At first, doctors could see that the DASH eating plan worked, but they did not understand how. Then researchers found that the diet appears to have the same effect on the body as diuretic medications (water pills) that help remove excess water the body retains. Diuretics are routinely prescribed for treating high blood pressure. Because sodium (salt) in foods tends to make the body retain water, the low-sodium component of the DASH diet may be a key factor in lowering blood pressure. Blood pressure reductions often begin to appear two weeks after starting the DASH eating plan. Even people with normal blood pressure can reduce their blood pressure further under the plan.

The DASH diet is based on a 2,000-calorie-a-day eating plan, so it is not strictly a weight-loss diet. But to reduce your calorie intake you can easily substitute lower-calorie foods for some that are recommended on the DASH diet. This tactic, combined with a boost in your physical activity, can be enough to help you shed some of those unwanted pounds over time. For example, eating a medium apple instead of four shortbread cookies for dessert will augment your fruit intake while significantly reducing your calorie intake. The chart below shows the daily recommendations for a typical 2,000-calorie DASH diet plan. Adjust your servings per day according to your calorie intake.

DASH RECOMMENDATIONS

Food	Servings Per Day
Grains (bread, cereal, pasta, rice)	7 to 8
Vegetables	4 to 5
Fruits	4 to 5
Low-fat or fat-free dairy products	2 to 3
Meat, poultry, fish	2 or less
Nuts, seeds, cooked dried beans	4 to 5 per week
Fats and oils*	2 to 3
Sweets**	5 per week

*Examples of fats and oils include 1 teaspoon of soft margarine or 1 tablespoon of salad dressing or mayonnaise.
**Examples of sweets include 1 tablespoon of sugar, jam, jelly, or pancake syrup, or 8 ounces of lemonade.

The DASH diet provides evidence for the strong influence that dietary sodium can have on blood pressure. Most of the salt in your diet comes not from the salt shaker but from the sodium that food manufacturers add during processing. Most packaged and processed foods are laden with sodium. One cup of packaged rice pilaf or macaroni and cheese, for example, can contain about 600 milligrams of sodium, which is 25 percent of the 2,300-milligram recommended daily allowance. One tablespoon of reduced-sodium soy sauce contains about 550 milligrams of sodium, or 23 percent of the daily allowance, while the same amount of regular soy sauce with twice the amount of sodium (1,100 milligrams) provides 46 percent of the daily sodium allowance.

Following are some processed foods that contain high amounts of sodium:

- Canned vegetables
- Frozen vegetables with sauce
- Tomato juice

- Soy sauce and other condiments, such as ketchup and mustard
- Processed cheese
- Canned beans (rinsing the beans removes a lot of the salt)
- Canned soups and broths
- Ham and other smoked meats
- Bologna and other sandwich meats
- Canned fish
- Frozen dinners
- Frozen pizza
- Some breakfast cereals
- Bread

Reading Food Labels: A Healthy Habit

Reading food labels can help you choose foods that are better for you. Labels on packaged food contain a section titled "Nutrition Facts," which lists important information, such as:

- Serving size
- Calorie content
- Fat and cholesterol content
- Sodium (salt) content
- Total carbohydrate content and the amounts of fiber and sugar
- Protein content
- Some vitamins and minerals

The serving size and the number of servings in the package are the keys to the nutrient breakdown for that food. The size of the serving determines the number of calories and the content of all the other nutrients on the label. In other words, if the label says a food has 12 grams of total fat, it means 12 grams in *one* serving. If the package contains three servings and you consume them all in one sitting, you will have eaten 3 × 12 grams, or 36 grams of fat.

It's especially important to check the fat, cholesterol, sugar, and sodium content. These are the nutrients that people often consume in excess. Make sure that foods you are thinking about buying contain minimal amounts of these nutrients. If the label says that the food contains trans fats, don't buy it. Trans fats have been found to be the most harmful kind of dietary fat.

Now look at the fiber (which is part of the "total carbohydrate" count) and vitamin and mineral contents. These are nutrients you need to eat more of. On the right side of the label, you will see a column called "% Daily Value." This column tells you whether a food is high or low in a particular nutrient so you can tell which nutrients contribute a lot or a little to your daily recommended allowance. For example, if you look at the label on a carton of milk, you will see that one serving supplies 30 percent of your daily recommended intake of calcium. Keep in mind that the percent daily values are based on recommendations for a 2,000-calorie diet, so if your calorie allotment is higher or lower, you will need to adjust the percentage the given nutrient represents in your diet. For more about how to read food labels, see page 66.

Instead of always relying on convenience foods, buy fresh foods whenever you can, or buy reduced-sodium or "no salt added" canned and processed foods. Cook foods without adding salt. Instead, use herbs and spices to add flavor to the dishes you serve. You can find out exactly how much salt is contained in packaged foods by learning to read food labels. Look for foods with less than 140 milligrams per serving, or 5 percent of the "daily value" for sodium.

9

Your Exercise Regimen

Physical activity is an essential component of your diabetes-management plan. Exercise improves blood sugar control, boosts heart health, promotes weight loss, reduces blood pressure, and makes you look and feel better. These benefits apply to anyone with type 2 diabetes—even people who have had diabetes for a long time and who may already have developed some complications from it. Regular exercise helps stabilize blood glucose levels by improving the body's use of insulin and by burning extra body fat, which improves the cells' sensitivity to insulin. Exercise also helps manage diabetes risks by increasing muscle mass and strength (muscle burns more calories than fat) and reducing blood pressure. An added benefit: exercise enhances bone density and strength, improving your ability to carry out everyday tasks.

The Pre-Exercise Physical Exam

Before you begin any exercise program, especially if you have been inactive for some time, make an appointment to see your doctor. Tell your doctor what type of exercise you plan to do and how often you plan to do it so he or she can adjust your meal plan or medication dosage if necessary. Before giving you the go-ahead to exercise, your doctor will perform a thorough physical examination and may order some laboratory tests. The doctor will also perform screenings for circulation and nerve problems that could affect your legs and feet during exercise. These screenings, collectively called a neurological evaluation, can be done in the doctor's office.

If your doctor detects nerve or blood vessel damage, he or she may advise you to avoid running, jogging, prolonged walking, and step exercises because these activities can cause muscle and joint injuries. Instead, your doctor might recommend swimming, biking, rowing, arm exercises, and other activities that don't require you to bear weight on your legs and feet.

If you are over age 35, or have heart disease, blood vessel problems, or nerve problems, your doctor will probably ask you to have an exercise stress test (see page 170). In addition to measuring your tolerance for exercise, an exercise stress test can identify an abnormal heart rate, blood pressure that rises too high during exercise, and previously undiagnosed heart disease. People who already have heart disease—diagnosed or undiagnosed—risk making it worse with overly vigorous exercise, resulting in chest pain called angina, abnormal heartbeat, or heart attack.

WARNING!

Exercise-Induced Retinal Detachment

In people who have diabetic retinopathy, the retina can be injured during jarring activities such as running and jumping when strands of scar tissue pull the retina loose from its normal position at the back of the eye. Retinal detachment can cause significant vision loss if left untreated. If you experience any of the following symptoms of retinal detachment during exercise or at any other time, call an ophthalmologist or go to a hospital emergency department immediately:

- A veil, shadow, or curtain obstructing your peripheral (side) vision
- Flashes of light
- A sudden shower of floaters that look like spots, insects, or spiderwebs
- Wavy or watery-looking vision
- A sudden reduction in vision

Early treatment for a detached retina can greatly improve your chances of saving your vision. An eye surgeon can treat retinal detachment with laser surgery (using high-energy light beams to reattach the retina to the back of the eye), cryotherapy (which freezes the retina into position), or, in some cases, with silicone oil (which is injected into the back of the eye to hold the retina in place while it heals).

Your doctor may also refer you to an ophthalmologist (eye doctor) for a dilated retinal examination to check for the presence of diabetic retinopathy (see page 183), a serious eye disorder that is common in people with diabetes. During vigorous exercise involving running or jumping or while lifting heavy weights, people who have diabetic retinopathy can damage the retina (the light-sensitive tissue that lines the back of the eye). The two most common eye injuries are retinal hemorrhage (bleeding from a rupture of the tiny blood vessels in the retina) and retinal detachment (in which the retina separates from the inner wall of the eye; see box).

Your doctor will probably tell you to closely monitor your feet for blisters and other minor irritations that could turn into major foot sores that are slow to heal. Wearing the right shoe for your activity (see page 81) is very important for preventing foot problems, especially if you have nerve or blood vessel damage. Many doctors recommend wearing shoes that have silica gel or air midsoles, which provide greater flexibility. Wearing polyester or polyester-cotton blend socks can help prevent blisters and keep feet dryer than 100 percent cotton socks.

Your doctor can help you select an appropriate activity to start with—usually brisk walking or swimming—to reduce your risk of exercise-induced complications such as a sudden lowering of blood sugar (hypoglycemia; see page 159). No matter which activity you choose, you will have to engage in it at a moderate pace for at least 30 to 60 minutes on most—preferably all—days of the week to get the most health benefits. Gradually work up to your maximum minutes of activity each day. Once your pre-exercise physical is complete and your doctor gives you the okay to exercise, you probably won't need to have your doctor monitor your exercise program regularly, unless you are injured.

WARNING!
Exercise Precautions

If you feel weak, dizzy, faint, nauseated, or short of breath, or have chest pain or tightness, don't ignore these symptoms, hoping they will go away on their own. The same goes for pain in your arm or jaw or heart palpitations. Stop exercising immediately. Chest pain and tightness or pain in an arm or jaw may signal a heart attack. If the pain doesn't go away in a minute or two, get emergency medical help.

If you feel symptoms of hypoglycemia coming on, consume fast-acting carbohydrates (which quickly raise blood glucose)—such as a piece of hard candy, 4 to 6 ounces of fruit juice, or five or six saltines—and see if you feel better. If your condition doesn't improve right away, seek medical help.

Getting Started

Most doctors tell people who are just starting to exercise to begin walking for 10 minutes at a time most days of the week at a leisurely pace. Work up to walking briskly for at least 30 minutes a day most days of the week. Brisk walking isn't just a stroll—it's striding quickly as if you were late for work or trying to catch a bus. Walking briskly, you should cover about 1½ miles in half an hour. As your fitness improves, you can add other activities such as swimming, biking, cross-country skiing, or aerobic dancing to your routine to minimize boredom. Tennis, racquetball, soccer, and basketball are also excellent aerobic activities and have the added benefit of getting you involved with other people in a team or competitive effort. Also, having an exercise "buddy" increases the likelihood that you'll stick with it. But remember to perform moderately intense activities that do not overtax your heart, especially when you are just starting out. Aim for a target heart rate of 60 to 70 percent of your maximum heart rate. (See page 77 to find your target heart rate.)

If you don't have high blood pressure or the eye disorder diabetic retinopathy (see page 183), you should also engage in strength-building exercises (page 72). Strengthening exercises are especially good for people with type 2 diabetes because they can help you keep your blood sugar levels under control. People with diabetes who regularly lift weights or do other types of resistance exercise can reduce their blood sugar much more than those who try to control blood sugar with diet alone. Strength training helps your cells become more sensitive to insulin by improving your muscles' ability to absorb sugar from the blood. Strength training is also good for the heart, making it stronger and more efficient. And strength-building exercise helps offset the decline in muscle strength that can come with aging.

To begin strength training, do a variety of resistance activities that work most of your major muscle groups. Include exercises that bend and extend your hips, knees, ankles, shoulders, and elbows against weight. Start with one to three sets of 8 to 15 repetitions for each muscle group. Don't hold any contraction for more than 5 or 6 seconds to avoid putting too much stress on your heart. When you lift weights, avoid lifting extremely heavy loads because heavy lifting can make your blood pressure suddenly spike upward.

You don't have to go to a gym to use weight-training equipment. You can exercise the same muscles and joints using elastic bands, inner tubes, cuff weights, hand weights, or even canned foods or water-filled milk jugs. You can also do sit-ups, push-ups, pull-ups, lunges, and leg lifts, which set your body against its weight or against gravity. Do strength-training exercises at least twice a week for best results. Skip a day between resistance exercising to give your muscles a chance to rest and repair themselves.

If you exercise with a friend, tell the person you are with that you have type 2 diabetes and let him or her know what to do if you feel the symptoms of low blood sugar coming on. This is especially important if you are taking insulin. Hypoglycemia isn't the only complication that can occur during exercise. If you have heart disease, you could begin having chest pain (angina) or an irregular heartbeat—in an extreme situation, you could have a heart attack. Avoiding overly vigorous activity, especially at first, can prevent such harmful effects on your heart. But just to be safe, always let family and friends know where you will be when you exercise and how long you plan to exercise. It's a good idea to wear a diabetes medical identification bracelet or shoe tag while you exercise. Carrying a cell phone may also be a good idea, so you can call for help if you need to.

One way to avoid problems during physical activity, especially if the weather is hot, is to stay hydrated. Dehydration can adversely affect both your blood sugar levels and the function of your heart. Drink about two 8-ounce glasses of water in the 2 hours before you start exercising and then drink some water during and after exercise if you are thirsty. You don't need to drink sports drinks with electrolytes unless you are competing in or training for a marathon or other high-intensity activity that lasts for a long time. Most sports drinks contain a lot of sugar, which can affect blood glucose. Water is always the best choice.

Staying Motivated

As good as it is for you, exercise can sometimes get boring. That's why it's so important to develop strategies that will get you through the difficult times. Exercise needs to become a habit, like checking your blood sugar. The more consistent you are in the beginning, the more likely you are to continue with your new activity. The following steps can help you make exercise a lifetime habit:

- **Set aside time for exercise.** Stake out a time each day for working out, and don't let anything get in the way. Pick the time of day that is most convenient for you.
- **Maximize your comfort.** Wear loose clothes and shoes that fit properly. In bad weather, walk briskly in an indoor, climate-controlled mall instead of jogging outside.
- **Choose activities you enjoy.** If you like group activities, take a Pilates class or a step class or join a bike club.
- **Spread the news.** Tell your family and friends what time you exercise and ask them not to interrupt you when you are exercising. Better yet, get them to join you.
- **Make an exercise date.** Your kids have their playdates. Why not make an exercise date with a neighbor once a week or even more often? It will benefit you both, both physically and socially.
- **Set goals.** Make goals that are easy to achieve in the beginning—walking ½ mile a day, for example—so you feel that you are accomplishing something. Gradually increase your time and pace until you reach your target heart rate (see page 77). Reward yourself when you attain each new goal.
- **Change your routine.** Alternate jogging, biking, walking, swimming, and other exercises to keep from getting bored.
- **Don't think about it too much.** Try not to indulge in negative thinking about exercise: *I'm too tired; I'm too old; I just don't feel like it.* Get off the couch, put on your walking shoes, and get moving.
- **Expect to reach plateaus.** Don't give times when you fail to exercise too much importance. Think, *In spite of this setback, my overall exercise plan is a success.*

Managing Stress

Your response to stressful situations can affect your blood sugar. Being under pressure may cause you to neglect your diabetes-management program. You stop exercising, go back to your poor eating habits, forget to check your blood sugar levels regularly, or drink too much alcohol. Stress triggers the release of hormones such as adrenaline and cortisol, which normally raise blood sugar to provide energy to meet normal everyday challenges. But when stress is chronic and severe, the normally helpful hormones can contribute to insulin resistance (see page 12), cause blood glucose to fluctuate, and trigger the accumulation of fat deposits around the abdomen. Carrying a lot of weight in the abdomen makes the cells less sensitive to insulin. Abdominal fat is also a risk factor for heart disease, which often accompanies type 2 diabetes. To cope better with stress, try these techniques:

- **Do deep breathing exercises.** Periodically throughout the day, stop what you're doing for a few seconds, make your mind blank, and take three deep breaths. Your heart rate and blood pressure will drop and you'll feel better.

- **Get moving.** You will improve your mood along with your health.

- **Do yoga.** The full-body stretching and meditative state inspired by yoga will calm your body and mind.

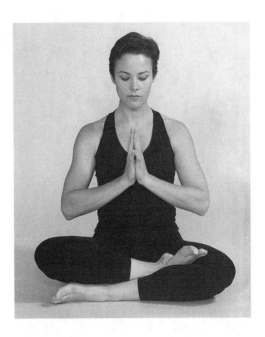

- **Meditate.** Ten to 20 minutes of quiet reflection can get you more in touch with your body as you sense each part of your body from head to toes.

- **Stay positive.** Stewing over a problem will just make you feel worse. Replace negative thoughts about a stressful situation with positive ones. Concentrate on the good things in your life.

- **Get a massage.** Ask your spouse or a friend for a back rub or get a full-body massage at a health club or a spa.

- **Make time for yourself.** Listen to some favorite music, work on your hobby, or relax in a warm bath.

- **Be flexible.** Don't make excessive demands on coworkers, employees, or family members. Think of alternative ways of finishing a task. Delegate responsibility.

- **Laugh.** Laughter, it seems, may lower blood pressure, reduce stress hormones, and boost the immune system.

10
Medication and Blood Sugar Testing

If diet, exercise, and weight loss fail to control your blood sugar, your doctor will probably prescribe a diabetes medication. When your doctor prescribes medication for your diabetes, he or she will tell you how, when, and how often to take it. Don't be reluctant to ask your doctor questions about each medication you are taking. The more you know about your treatment regimen, the more likely you are to follow your doctor's recommendations, maintain strict regulation of your blood glucose, and feel more in control of your health. Your doctor will teach you how to perform blood sugar testing so you can monitor your glucose levels on a regular basis—an important part of your diabetes care.

Diabetes Medications

If healthy eating, exercise, and losing weight don't reduce your blood glucose enough, you may have to take one or more types of diabetes medication. Although your body is making some insulin, it is not enough to meet the increased demands resulting from your cells' insensitivity to insulin. Your doctor will determine the best medication and overall treatment plan for getting your glucose level back to normal.

When you start taking medication to reduce your blood sugar, you still have to eat right, stay physically active, and maintain a healthy weight. Diabetes medications can't take the place of your prescribed meal plan and physical activity recommendations. Medications are an additional tool to help you manage your blood sugar.

Sugar-Lowering Medications

In years past, other than insulin (see page 135), only one class of medications—the sulfonylureas—was available for treating type 2 diabetes. Over the last decade, several other types of diabetes medications have been developed. Most sugar-lowering medications (unlike insulin) are taken in pill form by mouth and are designed to lower blood sugar in a specific way. The exception is a newer drug called exenatide, which is injected under the skin like insulin. Most medications for diabetes fall into the following groups:

- **Sulfonylureas** These medications stimulate the pancreas to make more insulin. Examples: glyburide, glipizide, and glimepiride.

- **Biguanides** This class of medications lowers the amount of glucose made by the liver. Example: metformin.

- **Alpha-Glucosidase Inhibitors** Known as starch blockers, these medications slow the digestion of starches. Examples: acarbohydrateose and miglitol.

- **Thiazolidinediones** These insulin-sensitizers make the cells more sensitive to the effects of insulin. Examples: pioglitazone and rosiglitazone.

- **Meglitinides and D-Phenylalanine Derivatives** These medications help the pancreas make more insulin. Example: repaglinide.

- **Incretin Mimetics** Incretins are a group of hormones produced by the digestive tract during digestion that stimulate insulin secretion and limit the increase in blood glucose after meals. The first in this newer class of drugs, an injectable medication "mimics" and augments the action of the body's natural incretin hormones. Example: exenatide.

Combination medications are also available that blend two or more of the above medications for better blood sugar control. For example, a medication that stimulates your pancreas to make more insulin (a sulfonylurea) is often combined with one that lowers the amount of glucose your liver makes (metformin). Many other medications for diabetes are currently under development and are in the process of being tested for safety and effectiveness or are awaiting government approval. Oral forms of compounds that increase incretin levels by slowing the breakdown of naturally occurring incretins are some of the medications that are under investigation.

If the medication your doctor prescribes is not getting your glucose down sufficiently, your doctor may increase the dose or add another medication. In the past, with fewer sugar-lowering medications to choose from, doctors would next prescribe insulin injections if sugar-lowering pills weren't effective. A newer option is a medication called exenatide, the first in a class of drugs called incretin mimetics; you inject exenatide under the skin using a prefilled penlike device before morning and evening meals.

Exenatide may be effective for some people who are unable to control their blood glucose with one or more sugar-lowering oral medications. Exenatide helps control blood glucose by stimulating insulin production in response to elevated blood glucose, inhibiting the release of glucose-raising glucagon after meals, slowing the rate of nutrient absorption into the bloodstream, slowing digestion in the stomach, and reducing food intake (possibly producing a modest weight loss). Still, for some people with type 2 diabetes, insulin injections are the best treatment option.

Like all medications, diabetes medications have potential side effects. Following are the most common possible side effects of the various diabetes medications:

- **Sulfonylureas** Side effects include low blood sugar (hypoglycemia; see page 159), skin reactions, dark urine, stomach upset, and sun sensitivity.
- **Biguanides** Side effects include upset stomach, nausea, and mild diarrhea. These side effects sometimes go away as your body gets used to the medication over several weeks. In very rare cases, biguanides can cause lactic acidosis, a buildup of lactic acid (a by-product of energy production) in the cells and bloodstream that can be life threatening in people whose liver or kidneys are not working properly.
- **Alpha-Glucosidase Inhibitors** Side effects of these starch-blockers include intestinal gas, diarrhea, and abdominal pain.

- **Thiazolidinediones** Side effects of these insulin-sensitizers include headache, sinus inflammation, backache, fatigue, muscle aches, swelling or fluid retention, and anemia. They also may make birth-control pills less effective.

- **Meglitinides and D-Phenylalanine Derivatives** The most common side effect is hypoglycemia.

- **Incretin Mimetics** The most common side effect is nausea, which usually subsides over time. Hypoglycemia is also a possible side effect when they are taken with other sugar-lowering medications.

Many of these medications should not be taken by people with kidney or liver disease or type 1 diabetes or by people who drink alcohol excessively. Pregnant women and women who are planning a pregnancy should talk with their doctors about their diabetes medications because many of these medications have not been tested during pregnancy.

Metformin, which reduces the amount of glucose made by the liver, is very interesting to doctors and medical researchers because it has several "side effects" that are actually good for you. For example, metformin stimulates minor weight loss, which in itself can improve control of blood sugar. Metformin can also improve blood fats (lipids such as cholesterol and triglycerides; see page 94), which are often elevated in people with type 2 diabetes. Another benefit of metformin is that unlike some other diabetes medications, it does not cause blood glucose to get too low (as long as it is the only diabetes medicine you are taking). Metformin has also been shown to be effective in preventing or delaying type 2 diabetes in people with prediabetes (see page 14).

To make sure you get the most out of your diabetes medication, ask your doctor the following questions:

- When do I take the medication: before a meal, with a meal, or after a meal?

- How often should I take it?

- Should I take it at the same time every day?

- What should I do if I forget to take my medication?

- What side effects could I experience?

- What should I do if I experience any side effects?

Insulin

In some people with type 2 diabetes, the pancreas may no longer make enough insulin for their body's needs. In this case, your doctor will recommend that you start giving yourself insulin injections. Insulin has to be taken as an injection under the skin with a small, short needle. If you took insulin in a pill, your digestive system would break it down and digest it before it got into your bloodstream. The purpose of insulin therapy is to replace the body's natural insulin to keep blood sugar levels as close to normal as possible. Careful control of blood sugar can help prevent both the acute, short-term problems (see chapter 12), such as hyperglycemic hyperosmolar nonketotic syndrome and diabetic ketoacidosis, and long-term, chronic complications (see chapter 13), such as eye, kidney, and nerve damage or heart disease.

Insulin Preparations

Several types of insulin preparations are available that work at different rates and last for different amounts of time. Many people with diabetes take two types of insulin. Your doctor will determine which type or types of insulin to prescribe based on your lifestyle, your blood sugar level, and the experience of his or her other patients with certain forms of insulin. Following are the most commonly prescribed forms of insulin, how soon after injection they start working, when they are most effective after injection, and when they stop working.

HOW DIFFERENT TYPES OF INSULIN WORK

Type of Insulin	Begins Working	Is Most Effective	Stops Working
Rapid-acting: lispro, aspart, or glulisine	5 to 20 minutes after injection	45 minutes to 3 hours after injection	3 to 5 hours after injection
Inhaled insulin	10 to 20 minutes after inhalation	2 hours after inhalation	About 6 hours after inhalation
Short-acting: Regular (R) insulin	30 to 45 minutes after injection	2 to 5 hours after injection	5 to 8 hours after injection
Intermediate-acting: NPH (N) insulin	1 to 3 hours after injection	6 to 12 hours after injection	16 to 24 hours after injection
Long-acting: Ultralente (U) insulin	4 to 6 hours after injection	8 to 20 hours after injection	24 to 28 hours after injection
Very long-acting: glargine	1 hour after injection	Works evenly for 24 hours	24 hours after injection

Like your own insulin, the insulin you inject brings blood sugar down by moving glucose from the blood into the cells. Once inside the cells, glucose provides the energy the cells need to function. Taking insulin lowers your blood sugar whether you eat or not. Eating at the times your doctor recommends can help you keep your blood glucose at a steady level. You will learn to match your meal and exercise times to the time when each insulin dose you take starts to work. Most people with type 2 diabetes need at least two insulin shots a day to maintain blood glucose at normal levels. Some people need to take insulin three or four times a day.

You should take insulin 30 minutes before a meal if you take regular insulin alone or with a longer-acting insulin. If you take rapid-action insulin, you should take your injection right before you eat. The speed at which insulin works inside your body also depends on where you inject it, the type and amount of physical activity you engage in, the length of time between your insulin dose and physical activity, and your body's unique response to the insulin. There is no one insulin treatment plan that works best for everyone, and finding the one that is best for you may take some adjustments. Remember, while insulin controls blood sugar levels, it does not cure diabetes: you have to keep taking your insulin even when you feel good. Always talk to your doctor if you are having any insulin-related problems.

Certain sites on your body are better than others for injecting yourself with insulin. Insulin injected near the stomach works the fastest, while insulin injected into the thigh works the slowest. Insulin injected into your arm falls somewhere in the middle. Doctors usually advise people with diabetes to rotate their insulin injection sites so the skin in a given area doesn't get too sore. Whatever insulin-injecting method you use, you still need to check your blood glucose level on a regular basis.

Ask your doctor to show you the correct way to inject insulin and which parts of your body are the best injection sites. These are the most common insulin-injection methods:

- **Syringes** Most people inject insulin with a syringe that delivers the insulin just under the skin. A syringe is a small hypodermic needle with a very sharp point attached to a hollow plastic tube that has a plunger inside.

- **Insulin Pens** The insulin pen looks like a cartridge pen, but it's filled with insulin instead of ink. Some pens use a refillable cartridge, while others are disposable. A thin, short needle sits at the end of the pen. To use the insulin pen, you turn a dial to the required dose of insulin, insert the needle under your skin, and press down a plunger to inject the insulin. Insulin pens are good for injecting very small, precise doses of insulin.

- **Jet Injectors** High-pressure jet injectors have no needles. Instead, they employ high-pressured air to send a fine spray of insulin through the skin. Jet injectors may cause less pain than syringes, but they are too expensive for most people to use routinely.

- **Insulin Pumps** These are used primarily by people who have type 1 diabetes, although some people with type 2 diabetes use an insulin pump to deliver a continuous dose of insulin. Worn on the outside of the body, the insulin pump connects to a catheter (a flexible tube) implanted in tissue under the skin of the abdomen. You can preset the pump to administer a constant, small dose of insulin, and use it to give yourself additional amounts of insulin at meal and snack times. When adjusted properly, insulin pumps can provide tight control of insulin levels, resulting in stable blood glucose.

Proper storage of insulin is important because excessive heat or cold breaks down the hormone, rendering it ineffective. Keep the bottle of insulin you are using at room temperature. Don't store it in the freezer or in very hot places, such as by a sunny window or in the glove compartment of your car. If you will not use an entire bottle of insulin within 30 days, store it in the refrigerator. Insulin kept at room temperature for more than 30 days should be thrown out. Keep at least one bottle of extra insulin in the refrigerator at all times as a backup. If your normally clear insulin looks cloudy, clumped, or crystallized; was exposed to very hot or cold temperatures; or has passed the expiration date, throw the bottle away and open a new one.

Insulin's Possible Side Effects

Like all medications, insulin has potential side effects. The most common side effect from insulin is low blood sugar (hypoglycemia; see page 159). Some diabetes medications, including sulfonylureas, meglinitides, D-phenylalanine derivatives, and combination medications, can also cause blood sugar to fall too low. Hypoglycemia can occur for a number of reasons, including delaying or skipping a meal, eating too little at a meal, getting more physical activity than usual, or taking too much insulin or other diabetes medication. Drinking alcohol can also lower blood sugar. You should suspect that your blood sugar is too low if you experience light-headedness, extreme hunger, tremors, confusion, and clammy sweating. If you think your blood glucose may be low, test it. If it is at or below 70 mg/dL, consume one of the following foods, which supplies about 15 grams of carbohydrate:

- ½ cup of fruit juice
- 8 ounces of milk
- 1 to 2 teaspoons of table sugar, honey, or pancake syrup
- ½ cup of soda pop
- Five or six pieces of hard candy
- Glucose gel or tablets, according to package directions for 15 grams of carbohydrate

Test your blood sugar again in 15 minutes. If it is still under 70 mg/dL, consume another 15 grams of carbohydrate. Then check your glucose again in 15 minutes. If your glucose is not low but you don't plan to eat your next meal for at least an hour, have a snack that combines starch and protein, such as cheese or peanut butter with crackers, half a meat sandwich, or a bowl of cereal with 1 cup of milk.

Some people experience redness, swelling, and itching at the injection site when they first start taking insulin. This condition usually clears up in a few days or weeks, but talk to your doctor about it as soon as you notice it. In very rare cases, people have a life-threatening, generalized allergic reaction to insulin. This reaction, called anaphylaxis, produces a rash over the whole body, shortness of breath, wheezing, low blood pressure, a fast pulse, or sweating, and can be fatal if not treated immediately. Call 911 or your local emergency number if you have a generalized reaction to insulin.

Inhaled Insulin

An inhaled form of human insulin is now available for treating diabetes. It is in the form of a fine, dry powder that is breathed into the lungs through the mouth using a specially designed inhalation device. Inhaled insulin has a rapid onset of action, is short-acting, and can be used alone or in conjunction with sugar-lowering medication or longer-acting insulin injections.

As with any insulin product, low blood sugar can be a side effect of inhaled insulin, so if you are taking it, you still need to carefully monitor your blood sugar. Other side effects include a cough, shortness of breath, sore throat, and dry mouth. You cannot use inhaled insulin if you smoke or if you have quit smoking within the last six months, or if you have asthma, bronchitis, or emphysema. While you are taking inhaled insulin you will have regular lung function tests to make sure the medication is not causing any lung problems.

> ## Intensive Insulin Treatment
>
> Some people with type 2 diabetes may need to consider intensive insulin treatment to maintain optimal blood sugar control. This therapy requires more frequent testing of blood glucose and three or more insulin injections throughout the day or the use of an insulin pump (see page 137). If you are considering intensive insulin treatment, ask your doctor if it is an option for you.

Checking Your Blood Sugar

Regularly checking blood sugar levels is a routine and essential part of diabetes management. Blood sugar testing at home helps you evaluate how well your food intake, exercise, and medication regimen are working to control your blood sugar levels. The closer to normal your blood sugar is, the less likely you are to develop serious chronic complications such as heart disease, nerve damage, and kidney failure.

How to Check Your Blood Sugar

Most people with type 2 diabetes check their blood sugar level with test strips and a portable glucose meter, a small, battery-powered device that measures the amount of sugar in a small sample of blood taken from a fingertip. This test is commonly known as a fingerstick test. To test your blood sugar using a glucose meter, you place a small drop of blood from your fingertip on a disposable test strip (which is coated with chemicals that blend with the glucose in your blood) and put the strip in the meter. Glucose meters differ in speed, size, cost, the amount of blood needed for each test, and the capacity to store test results in memory. The meter displays the glucose level as a number expressed in milligrams per deciliter (mg/dL). Some meters are easier to read than others. Some new models can record and store several consecutive test results, and some can connect to a personal computer to download the test results and print them out.

Nondiabetic vs. Diabetic Blood Sugar Levels

Following are the normal ranges for blood glucose in people who do not have diabetes and the target blood glucose ranges for people who have diabetes. Checking your blood glucose as often as your doctor recommends and maintaining your glucose within these target ranges can keep you healthy and reduce your risk of complications.

Normal Blood Sugar Ranges in People Who Do Not Have Diabetes

Upon waking (fasting)	70 to 100 mg/dL
After a meal	70 to 140 mg/dL

Target Blood Sugar Ranges in People with Diabetes

Before meals	90 to 130 mg/dL
1 to 2 Hours after the start of a meal	Less than 180 mg/dL
Hypoglycemia (low blood sugar)	50 to 60 mg/dL or below

People usually decide which glucose meter to use based on the cost, ease of use, size, and accuracy. Your doctor or diabetes educator will teach you how to use the meter that you choose. It's important to bring your glucose meter with you to your doctor's office so he or she can watch you take a reading and make sure you are using the meter correctly. Have your meter calibrated against a laboratory reading every few months to maintain its accuracy.

Self-checking of blood sugar is beneficial for everyone with diabetes, but it is especially important for people who take insulin. Some people need to test their blood sugar more frequently than others. Your doctor will recommend the exact frequency of your blood sugar testing. Some of the key times that you may be asked to test are before meals, 1 or 2 hours after meals, at bedtime, occasionally at 3:00 A.M., and any time you experience a feeling of low blood sugar. You should test more often when you start taking a new medication or when you are ill or under more stress than usual.

What Causes High Blood Sugar Readings?

A high blood sugar level is a reading higher than 180 mg/dL 2 hours after eating or 130 mg/dL before eating. Talk to your doctor to find out what he or she thinks is a prudent blood sugar target for you both before and after meals. High blood sugar levels can be affected by many factors, including:

- Overeating
- Lack of exercise
- Insufficient sugar-lowering medication or insulin
- A spoiled batch of insulin
- Illness, infection, injury, or surgery
- An inaccurate blood glucose meter

Blood sugar levels that stay high for long periods can put you at risk for long-term complications such as eye disease, kidney disease, nerve damage, and heart disease. Call your doctor immediately if your blood sugar has been over 240 mg/dL for longer than a day. You should also call your doctor right away if you have more than just a small amount of ketones in your urine (produced when an insufficiency of insulin forces the body to break down fat to produce energy) for more than a few hours or if you have any symptoms of ketoacidosis (see page 163) such as unusual sleepiness, weakness, extreme thirst, frequent urination, leg cramps, or nausea.

11

Experimental Treatments and Special Situations

Many new, experimental treatments for type 2 diabetes are being developed. This chapter discusses some of these promising new treatments, such as beta cell regeneration and pancreas transplants, and covers alternative therapies for diabetes treatment—those that fall outside traditional Western medical practice. You will also learn some helpful tips for what to do in special situations, such as when you are ill or are traveling. Finally, if you are a woman with diabetes who is pregnant, you will find reassuring advice about how to keep your blood glucose under control to ensure that you have a healthy pregnancy.

Experimental Treatments for Type 2 Diabetes

Each year, more and more people with diabetes turn to experimental treatments. But before trying an experimental treatment, discuss it with your doctor. Ask about the treatment's safety and effectiveness and whether it could interact or interfere with your diabetes medications or any other medications you are taking or treatment you are undergoing.

Pancreas Transplants

Pancreas transplantation has become a widely used treatment for people with type 1 diabetes who have kidney disease requiring a kidney transplant or who are incapacitated with severe, frequent hypoglycemia. Pancreas transplants remain experimental for other people with type 1 diabetes and for people with type 2 diabetes because of the significant side effects of the immune-suppressing medications that a person with a transplant must take for life to prevent organ rejection. The supply of available donor pancreases is small. Few people with type 2 diabetes lose so much of their capacity to make insulin that they would qualify for a pancreas transplant, and because people with type 2 diabetes are insulin resistant (insensitive to the effects of insulin), their need for insulin may be greater than a transplanted pancreas could supply.

Islet Cell Transplants

Some researchers are studying alternatives to whole pancreas transplants and are testing the possibility of transplanting clusters of cells called islets that reside inside the pancreas. These islet clusters contain two types of cells: alpha cells, which make glucagon (a hormone that raises the level of sugar in the blood) and beta cells (which manufacture insulin). Insulin-producing beta cells make up only about 2 percent of the pancreas. In an experimental procedure called islet transplantation, islets are taken from a donor pancreas and transferred into the liver of a person with diabetes. Once implanted, the beta cells in these islets start to make and release insulin. If islet transplantation is found to be safe and effective, it would be a desirable treatment option for people with diabetes because transplanting islet cells is simpler than the complicated surgery required to transplant a whole pancreas.

However, some major issues need to be resolved before islet transplantation becomes a widespread treatment. One issue is the uncertainty over where to transplant the islets; in the experimental trials, they are being injected into the liver. Also, getting a sufficient number of islets for one successful transplant requires the use of two or more donor pancreases. Because of the shortage of donor pancreases, this procedure is currently performed only in a small number of people with type 1 diabetes. People with type 2 diabetes require more insulin-producing islet cells than people with type 1 because their cells are resistant to the effects of insulin, which increases their need for insulin.

In addition, the antirejection, immune-suppressing drugs that are required after a transplant can affect the transplanted islet cells, eventually causing them to lose their capacity to produce insulin. To overcome the need for immune-suppressing drugs to avoid rejection after islet cell transplantation, researchers are looking for ways to "disguise" the transplanted cells (such as by encapsulating them) to prevent the immune system from attacking them. Other studies are looking into using islet cells from pigs for transplants to overcome the shortage of available human islets.

Beta Cell Regeneration

Coaxing other cells in the pancreas into becoming insulin-producing beta cells could some day be an effective alternative to pancreas and islet cell transplants. As the body becomes resistant to insulin, it demands more and more insulin in an attempt to compensate for the loss of the cells' sensitivity. The beta cells initially churn out increasing amounts of insulin, but they eventually become overtaxed by the high demand and begin to fail. Beta cell regeneration seeks to replenish the supply of beta cells in order to restore insulin production in the pancreas.

Programming Non–Beta Cells to Produce Insulin

Another experimental approach for treating diabetes is to manipulate the genes of some cells in the body that are not beta cells to produce and secrete insulin in response to glucose levels in the blood. One study is seeking to genetically engineer liver cells to produce insulin that can be readily released into the bloodstream; this research uses the natural glucose and insulin response mechanisms in the liver that stimulate insulin production when blood glucose is high and suppress it when blood sugar is low.

Stem-Cell Research

Stem cells are primitive cells that have the ability to multiply and become specific types of cells. Researchers are using several approaches for isolating and growing stem cells or islet precursor cells from fetal and adult pancreatic tissue, including the cells that line the pancreatic ducts. Other researchers are investigating ways to grow and coax embryonic stem cells into becoming insulin-producing islet cells of the pancreas. Theoretically, with a supply of available stem cells, a line of embryonic stem cells could be grown up as needed for anyone requiring a transplant; before being transplanted, these cells could be engineered to avoid rejection, eliminating the need for immune-suppressing drugs.

Before this therapy can be used in people, researchers will need to rule out the possibility that precursor or stemlike cells transplanted into the body could revert to a primitive state from which they could develop into any type of cell and then multiply and form tumors. Also, the process of producing human embryonic stem cells remains controversial because of the ethical issues raised over using human embryos for research. Currently, the federal government has restricted its funding to the use of embryonic stem cell lines that have already been developed. However, researchers in the United States can continue to use other sources of funds to conduct independent research on newly developed lines of human embryonic stem cells.

Complementary and Alternative Therapies

Another area of research being explored for treating type 2 diabetes is the use of complementary or alternative therapies. Complementary medicine refers to treatments such as acupuncture that are used in addition to conventional treatments. Alternative therapies are those that generally lie outside traditional Western medicine. Some people who have type 2 diabetes use complementary or alternative therapies to try to improve their condition. Although some of these therapies may provide some improvement in blood glucose control, others are ineffective or even harmful. If you are thinking about using a complementary or an alternative medical procedure, always discuss it with your doctor first to find out if it is safe and effective.

A complementary or alternative therapy should not replace the treatment prescribed by your doctor and diabetes educator or dietitian. The US Food and Drug Administration (FDA) does not strictly regulate or standardize herbal or dietary supplements so there is no guarantee of their strength, purity, or safety. You should consider that taking an herbal remedy is like taking a medication that has not been approved by the FDA. In addition, herbal supplements can be expensive, can have side effects (which are not required to be listed on package inserts, as are side effects from regulated medications), and can interfere with medications you are taking.

Acupuncture

Acupuncture is a treatment in which a practitioner inserts needles into certain points on the skin, usually to provide relief from chronic pain. Acupuncture is sometimes used by people with type 2 diabetes who have painful nerve damage (see page 177). In some cases, the technique seems to be effective in relieving pain by generating the release of the body's natural painkillers (called endorphins).

Biofeedback

Biofeedback uses relaxation and stress-reduction techniques to help a person become more aware of and learn to control involuntary body functions such as heart rate and the body's response to pain. Guided imagery is a relaxation technique that is often used with biofeedback. Using guided imagery, a person focuses on peaceful mental images such as ocean waves, or images of his or her body curing a chronic disease such as diabetes. People using this technique sometimes find that these positive images can, at least temporarily, improve their condition.

Chromium

The benefit of adding increased amounts of the mineral chromium to the diets of people with diabetes has been studied and debated for many years. The body needs chromium to make glucose tolerance factor, a protein that helps improve the action of insulin. Although some studies have found that taking chromium supplements may improve blood sugar control in some people, doctors do not recommend chromium supplements for treating diabetes because of insufficient evidence of their safety and effectiveness.

Ginseng

Several types of plants are called ginseng, but most studies of ginseng and diabetes have used American ginseng, grown in Wisconsin. These studies have shown some blood-sugar-reducing effects after eating, as well as reductions in A1C levels (average blood glucose levels over a three-month period; see page 92). Asian ginseng has been used for centuries in Chinese medicine to treat diabetes. Larger and more long-term studies are needed before doctors can consider recommending the use of ginseng supplements for type 2 diabetes. One major problem is that the amount of glucose-lowering compound in ginseng plants varies widely. Talk to your doctor before trying these supplements.

Magnesium

Research suggests that a deficiency of magnesium may worsen blood glucose control in people with type 2 diabetes. A deficiency of magnesium seems to interfere with insulin secretion in the pancreas and increase insulin resistance in muscle and fat cells. Two large studies have found that people who have a higher dietary intake of magnesium (through consumption of whole grains, nuts, and green leafy vegetables) have a decreased risk of developing type 2 diabetes. Evidence also suggests that an insufficiency of magnesium may contribute to some complications in people who have diabetes. Talk to your doctor if you are considering taking magnesium supplements.

Vanadium

Found in tiny amounts in plants and animals, the mineral vanadium may help normalize blood glucose levels by improving insulin sensitivity. Foods that supply vanadium include whole grains, dill, fish, olives, meat, and vegetables oils. Researchers are currently exploring how vanadium works in the body, looking for potential side effects, and trying to establish safe doses for supplements. Do not take vanadium supplements without talking to your doctor first.

Gingko Biloba

Gingko biloba has antioxidant, anti-inflammatory, and nerve-protecting properties that may be useful in preventing and treating early-stage nerve damage caused by diabetes. But, as with all supplements, talk to your doctor if you are considering taking gingko biloba.

Indian Kino

Indian kino is a gummy tree resin that has long been used for treating diabetes in India, where it is thought to prevent damage to and even regenerate the beta cells in the pancreas that produce insulin. However, no studies have been done in the United States to prove these effects, and doctors are doubtful about these claims.

Bitter Melon

In Asia, Africa, and South America, the extract of this tropical fruit is used as a folk remedy for diabetes. However, the use of bitter melon for treating diabetes has not been studied in humans, and there is limited scientific evidence about its safety or effectiveness.

Diabetes Care at Special Times

Diabetes is a chronic condition that you will most likely have for the rest of your life. The success of your diabetes treatment depends on how well you adapt your lifestyle to improving your blood glucose control. Most important is how well you blend your activity level and diet to reach and maintain a healthy weight. Some situations—such as when you are sick, traveling, or pregnant (or even thinking about getting pregnant)—require extra precautions and effort to keep your blood sugar at a healthy level.

When You're Sick

If you have diabetes, you need to take especially good care of yourself when you have a cold, the flu, or any other infection or illness, because being sick can cause your blood sugar level to rise. In severe cases, extremely high glucose levels can result in a diabetic coma. To keep a minor health problem from becoming a serious condition, plan in advance what to do when you are sick. Keep extra medical supplies on hand to deal with an emergency.

When you get sick, your body is under a lot of stress. To cope with the added burden, your body sends out hormones to fight the illness. However, these normally helpful hormones can elevate blood sugar levels and block insulin's ability to reduce blood sugar. For this reason, being sick makes blood sugar more difficult to control. Rarely in people with type 2 diabetes, high blood sugar can lead to a serious condition called hyperglycemic hyperosmolar nonketotic syndrome (HHNS; see page 162). In extreme cases, HHNS can result in a form of diabetic coma.

To prepare in advance for the times when you are sick, keep the phone numbers of your doctor and diabetes educator or dietitian in a handy place near the phone. Ask them how you can reach them at night and on weekends and holidays. You don't have to call the doctor every time you sneeze, but there are certain times when you should call, including in the following situations:

- You have had a fever for two days and you aren't feeling better.
- You have vomited more than once.
- You have had diarrhea for longer than 6 hours.
- You tested your urine and found that you have moderate to large amounts of ketones in it.
- Your glucose level is over 240 even though you've taken extra insulin to lower it.
- You take sugar-lowering pills and your blood sugar has risen above 240 mg/dL before meals or has been that high for longer than a day.
- Your chest hurts, you are having trouble breathing, your breath smells fruity, you feel sleepier than usual, or your lips or tongue are dry and cracked. These symptoms could be a sign of ketoacidosis, dehydration, or another serious condition.
- You are unsure what to do to take care of yourself.

In general, when you are ill, if you take diabetes medication, you should keep taking it while you're sick even if you can't keep food down or you have been vomiting. Ask your doctor if you should change the dosage of your medicine. Home blood glucose testing remains very important when you are sick or under a lot of stress because it gives you the information you need to fine-tune your medication or insulin treatment to keep your blood sugar level from getting too high or too low. Here are some other tips to help you get through your illness:

- Test your blood sugar level every 4 hours and write it down so you can see if it changes over time.
- If you have a fever or diarrhea, drink at least 8 ounces of water or other sugar-free, caffeine-free drinks every hour you are awake.
- If you don't feel like eating, try drinking juice or eating crackers, frozen ice pops, or soup.
- If you can't keep food down at all, try drinking small amounts of clear liquids containing sugar, such as ginger ale. If you vomit more than two or three times, contact your doctor immediately.
- Test your urine for ketones if your blood glucose is over 240 mg/dL or if you can't keep food or liquids down. Call your doctor right away if you have moderate or large amounts of ketones in your urine on two consecutive tests.

When You're Traveling

When it comes to controlling your blood sugar, you can't take a holiday. When you're on a business trip or on vacation, you may be tempted to go off your meal plan or become lax about taking your medication. You may drink more alcohol than usual. But taking care of your diabetes is just as important when you are away as it is when you are at home.

Before going on a lengthy trip, see your doctor for a checkup to make sure your diabetes is under control. Make the appointment far enough in advance so you can get your diabetes under control if necessary before you leave. If you need to have any immunizations, get them at least one month before you depart so that if the shots make you sick you'll have time to recover fully before the trip.

Wear a medical identification bracelet or necklace that indicates that you have diabetes. If you're going to a country that has a different language, learn how to say "I have diabetes" and "I need sugar or fruit juice, please" in the local language. Here are some more tips to help ensure a safe trip and help you keep your blood sugar under control while you're away:

- Stick to your meal plan as much as you can when you eat out. Carry a snack with you in case you have to wait a long time to be served.

- Ask your doctor or diabetes educator in advance how much alcohol you can safely drink and limit your intake to that amount. Eat something when you drink alcohol.

- If you are taking a long car trip, check your blood glucose level before driving. If you take insulin, stop and check your blood sugar again every 2 hours. Bring along snacks such as fruit, crackers, juice, or soda in the car in case your blood sugar drops too low.

- If you are taking a plane, ask in advance about diabetic meals. Most airlines accommodate special dietary needs. Again, carry healthy snacks with you if there will be no meal served or in case meals are late.

- Keep your diabetes medication, insulin, and syringes in a carry-on bag; don't pack them in your checked baggage. The limit of one carry-on and one personal item (purse, briefcase, or computer case) does not apply to medical supplies or equipment. You can pack some extra supplies in your checked luggage.

- To avoid foot problems, take comfortable shoes that fit you well. Never go barefoot; wear flip-flops or slippers in your hotel room. Check your feet for redness, sores, and blisters every day.

- If you are going to a foreign country or will be away for a long time, ask your doctor for a written prescription for your diabetes medication.

- If you take insulin, buy an insulated bag to carry it in so it doesn't get too hot or too cold while traveling.

- Take extra supplies with you. Don't count on being able to buy extra supplies when you reach your destination; different countries use different kinds of insulin, syringes, test strips, and medications.

- Ask your doctor how to adjust your medication and insulin doses if you will be crossing time zones.

Always tell the security screeners at the airport that you have diabetes and that you are carrying your supplies with you. Ask your doctor in advance for a letter stating that you have diabetes and need to carry syringes so you can show it to the screener or to customs agents if you have to. The following diabetes-related supplies and equipment are allowed through airport security checkpoints once they have been screened:

- Clearly labeled insulin and insulin-loaded dispensing equipment (vials or a box of individual vials, jet injectors, pens, infusers, and preloaded syringes)
- An unlimited number of unused syringes, when accompanied by insulin or other injectable medication
- Lancets, blood glucose meters, blood glucose meter test strips, alcohol swabs, and meter-testing solutions
- Insulin pumps and insulin pump supplies (cleaning agents, batteries, plastic tubing, infusion kit, catheter, and needle)
- A glucagon emergency kit
- Urine ketone test strips
- An unlimited number of used syringes when carried in a "sharps" disposal container or other similar hard-surface container

Inform the screeners if you are wearing an insulin pump and explain that you cannot go through the metal detector or be hand-wanded while wearing it. Explain to the screener that the insulin pump cannot be removed because it is infusing life-saving insulin into your body. Insulin pumps and supplies have to be accompanied by insulin that has professionally printed labels clearly identifying it or with the manufacturer's name or pharmacy label visible. You always have the option of asking for visual inspection of your insulin and diabetes supplies. Be sure to tell the security screeners if you are experiencing low blood sugar and need medical help.

Don't forget to keep up your exercise regimen while you are away from home. Changing your level of physical activity could affect your blood sugar. Many hotels have fitness centers or agreements with local health clubs that allow hotel guests to use their facilities. Of course, walking is always an excellent option—you'll be active and you can see and enjoy the sights in the places you are visiting.

If You Have Diabetes and Become Pregnant

Planning ahead is crucial if you have diabetes and you want to get pregnant. Before you become pregnant, you will need to bring your blood glucose down into the normal range. High blood sugar levels during pregnancy can be dangerous for both you and your baby. You also face increased health risks such as high blood pressure or a worsening of any diabetic complications you already have, especially eye disease (diabetic retinopathy; see page 183).

During the first six to eight weeks of pregnancy, a fetus can develop birth defects if the mother's blood sugar is too high. High blood sugar can also cause miscarriage during the first trimester. During the later stages of pregnancy, elevated blood sugar levels can cause premature birth or stillbirth. Excess blood sugar can cause the fetus to grow larger than normal, making delivery more difficult. A baby can also be born with jaundice from an accumulation of old blood cells that the baby's liver can't dispose of fast enough.

If you plan to get pregnant, work with your doctor to get your blood glucose as close to normal as possible. Some medications are not safe to take during pregnancy. Your doctor may ask you to stop taking a particular medication or may prescribe another medication or treatment when you plan to get pregnant. Following these additional guidelines can help ensure a healthy pregnancy:

- Try to see an obstetrician who has experience taking care of pregnant women with diabetes.
- Have your eyes and kidneys checked because pregnancy can make eye and kidney problems worse.
- Don't smoke, drink alcohol, or use illegal drugs during your pregnancy.
- Closely follow the meal plan your doctor, diabetes educator, or dietitian has developed for you.

If you take insulin, your doctor will probably prescribe intensive insulin therapy (see page 139) as a way to help keep your blood sugar within the normal range. This therapy will involve frequent monitoring of your blood sugar using various types of insulin and regulation of your dosage based on your blood sugar levels, diet, and any changes in your daily routine. Your doctor will tell you what your blood sugar goal is, which may be lower than what it was before your pregnancy (because pregnancy itself normally lowers blood glucose).

If you have type 2 diabetes, you will probably stop taking the glucose-lowering pills your doctor prescribed and start taking insulin to control your blood sugar during your pregnancy. Intensive insulin therapy can give you greater control over your blood sugar levels. In addition, insulin is recommended during pregnancy because the safety of glucose-lowering medications for pregnant women and their fetuses is not known for sure.

Taking care of your diabetes while you are pregnant may seem like a lot of work, but the health rewards are high—for both you and your baby. If you are already pregnant, see your doctor right away. It's not too late to bring your blood sugar close to normal so you can stay healthy during the rest of your pregnancy. If you develop diabetes after you become pregnant, see chapter 15, which discusses gestational diabetes.

PART FOUR

Complications of Diabetes

12

Acute Complications

If you are unable to control your blood glucose levels, you may quickly end up with potentially serious medical problems. Fortunately, these acute complications can usually be prevented or reversed with prompt treatment. The three most common acute, or short-term, complications of type 2 diabetes are hypoglycemia (low blood sugar), hyperglycemic hyperosmolar nonketotic syndrome (HHNS), and diabetic ketoacidosis. Become familiar with the symptoms of each condition, so you can get medical help right away if you feel symptoms coming on.

Hypoglycemia

Hypoglycemia, also called low blood sugar, occurs when your blood sugar level falls too low. This means that your body, especially your brain, doesn't have enough fuel to function well. When blood glucose begins to drop, your pancreas releases a hormone called glucagon that instructs the liver to break down stored sugar (glycogen) and send it into the bloodstream. If you have diabetes, this process may not work very well, making it harder for blood sugar to return to normal. Mild hypoglycemia is fairly common among people with type 2 diabetes, but serious episodes are rare.

Hypoglycemia is more likely to occur when you are keeping tight control of your blood sugar level, so you need to be extra careful about not letting it slip into the danger zone. For example, low blood sugar can develop when you take your diabetes medication and fail to eat enough, or when you increase your physical activity, take too much medication, or drink too much alcohol.

In people with type 2 diabetes, hypoglycemia is usually mild and can be reversed by drinking or eating something sweet, such as orange juice or a piece of hard candy. But severe cases can cause loss of consciousness and even death. In extreme cases in which a person loses consciousness and can't eat, the glucose-raising hormone glucagon can be injected to raise blood sugar quickly. People who take insulin should keep a glucagon emergency kit at home for just such emergencies.

Warning Signs of Hypoglycemia

The signs of hypoglycemia can vary from person to person, so you should become familiar with your usual symptoms. You might have one or more of the following signs or symptoms of hypoglycemia, which can occur suddenly:

- Hunger
- Trembling
- Perspiration
- Feeling drunk
- Rapid heartbeat
- Dizziness or light-headedness
- Feeling sleepy
- Confusion
- Difficulty speaking
- Anxiety
- Weakness

Hypoglycemia can develop at night when you're asleep. When this occurs, you might cry out, have nightmares, or have night sweats. You may also feel tired, irritable, or confused when you wake up.

Describe your familiar symptoms to your family and friends so they can help you if your blood pressure gets too low. If your child has diabetes, tell the school staff about the possibility of hypoglycemia and what to do if your child has it. If you take a diabetes medication that can cause hypoglycemia, always carry a piece of hard candy or other sweet with you to quickly raise your blood glucose. Wearing a medical identification bracelet or necklace saying you have diabetes is a good idea for alerting people to your condition if you are unconscious and cannot communicate.

It is clearly vital to prevent yourself from having hypoglycemia while you are driving. Checking your blood sugar levels frequently and snacking between meals will help keep your blood sugar steady and help you avoid accidents.

If you develop hypoglycemia more often than once a week, talk to your doctor. You may need a change in your treatment plan—less medication, a different medication, an alteration in your diet, or an adjustment in your exercise regimen. You might need to have a snack or change your medication dose before engaging in unplanned exercise such as shoveling snow.

A Quick Fix for Hypoglycemia

If you have a feeling that your blood sugar level is too low, quickly check it with your blood glucose meter (see page 139). If your blood sugar is 70 mg/dL or lower, consume one of the following foods right away to raise it:

- ½ cup of fruit juice
- ½ cup of a sugary soft drink (not diet or sugar-free)
- 1 cup of milk
- 5 or 6 pieces of hard candy
- 1 or 2 teaspoons of sugar or honey
- 2 or 3 glucose tablets

After 15 minutes, check your blood sugar level again to make sure it is still not too low. If it's still low, have another serving of something sweet. Repeat these steps until your blood glucose rises above 70 mg/dL. Then, if you don't plan to have a meal for the next hour or more, have a snack.

ACUTE COMPLICATIONS   161

Preventing Hypoglycemia

You can reduce your chances of having hypoglycemia by carefully planning when you eat and coordinating mealtimes and snacks with your glucose-lowering medication and exercise. The following steps can help you avoid hypoglycemia:

- Follow the meal plan provided by your doctor, diabetes educator, or dietitian.
- Space your meals evenly throughout the day and eat between-meal snacks.
- Make sure to eat your meals no more than 5 hours apart.
- Wait for half an hour to an hour after eating before exercising.
- Double-check the dose of your glucose-lowering medication before you take it to make sure you aren't taking too much.
- Carry a quick-fix food (see the previous page) such as hard candy with you at all times. Keep a sugar-carbohydrate-protein food (such as an energy bar) in your car in case your blood sugar gets too low while you are driving.
- Check your blood sugar level regularly throughout the day.
- Make sure a family member or a friend knows how to give you a glucagon injection if you become unconscious.

Hyperglycemic Hyperosmolar Nonketotic Syndrome

People with type 2 diabetes whose blood sugar levels rise extremely high are susceptible to a serious condition called hyperglycemic hyperosmolar nonketotic syndrome (HHNS). As your blood sugar soars, your body tries to eliminate the excess sugar through the urine. At first, your body makes lots of urine and you have to urinate frequently. Then you begin to get dehydrated and your urine becomes concentrated and dark. The dehydration gets worse over a period of days to weeks and, if not treated, can eventually lead to seizures, coma, and death.

HHNS usually occurs in people over the age of 60 and is most often triggered by an infection. It can also be triggered by some medications (such as diuretics and other heart medications or steroids) and some medical conditions (such as a bleeding ulcer, a blood clot, a heart attack, or kidney failure).

Symptoms of HHNS include intense thirst, increased urination, weakness, drowsiness, headache, restlessness, an altered mental state, or paralysis. If you experience any of these symptoms, test your blood sugar level immediately and call your doctor right away if it is 500 mg/dL or higher. You will probably have to go to the hospital, where you can receive intravenous (through a vein) fluids along with insulin to lower your blood sugar.

To prevent HHNS, test your blood glucose level regularly—every 4 hours when you are sick—and take extra-good care of yourself when you are ill.

Diabetic Ketoacidosis

Doctors used to see life-threatening diabetic ketoacidosis almost exclusively in people with type 1 diabetes, but now the incidence seems to be on the rise in people with type 2 diabetes, especially Hispanics and African Americans. The reason for the upsurge remains unclear. The underlying trigger for diabetic ketoacidosis is insufficient insulin. Ketoacidosis usually appears in response to something, such as a severe infection, that places added stress on the body, causing it to need more insulin than normal. Other possible contributing factors include alcohol abuse, an injury, a pulmonary embolism (a blood clot in the lung), or a heart attack.

Remember that when you have diabetes, even though your blood sugar levels may be high, your cells can't use the glucose for energy without insulin. Insulin also regulates the storage and release of fat from fat tissue. When insulin is severely lacking, or when a person is extremely resistant to insulin, fat release is increased. The by-products of the breakdown of fat are substances called ketone bodies, or ketones for short. The buildup of ketones in the blood is toxic at high levels, causing acidosis and dangerous irregularities in the organs, including the heart. Diabetic ketoacidosis usually develops gradually over several hours, but it is a medical emergency.

The most common symptoms of diabetic ketoacidosis are severe thirst, nausea and vomiting, rapid heartbeat, abdominal pain, drowsiness, and a fruity odor to the breath (produced by the ketones). A characteristic pattern of deep, rapid breathing punctuated by deep sighs (known medically as Kussmaul breathing) is a hallmark of diabetic ketoacidosis. Left untreated, the condition can progress to seizures, coma, and death. If you or someone you are with starts to develop this cluster of symptoms, call 911 immediately. At the hospital, you will receive replacement fluids, insulin, and potassium to restore the balance of electrolytes (essential minerals in the bloodstream that maintain the body's chemical balance).

You can avoid diabetic ketoacidosis by carefully following your diabetes management plan, which includes taking your diabetes medicine as directed by your doctor. You should also closely follow your meal plan and exercise regimen and check your blood sugar frequently. When you are ill, it is essential to call your doctor before symptoms progress to diabetic ketoacidosis.

13

Chronic Complications

Type 2 diabetes is a chronic disease that can cause serious chronic, or long-term, complications when blood sugar is not well-controlled. The most common chronic complications of type 2 diabetes are heart disease, nerve damage, blood circulation problems, eye damage, kidney disease, and dental problems. These conditions in turn can cause other serious health problems. For example, the combination of poor blood flow and nerve damage in the feet or legs can produce skin ulcers or infections that don't heal, sometimes resulting in amputation. Damage to blood vessels in the eyes can eventually cause blindness. Some of these diabetic complications have no symptoms in the early stages, but they all result from damage to blood vessels or nerves as a result of high blood sugar.

People with diabetes who keep their blood glucose levels within the normal range are far less likely to have long-term complications than those who don't maintain good control of their glucose. The number-one way to prevent, delay, or minimize most of the complications of diabetes is to carefully control your blood glucose. Good blood glucose control involves strictly following your treatment plan, which combines frequent medical checkups, a diabetes meal plan, regular exercise, maintaining a healthy weight, and strict control of your blood glucose.

Heart Disease

People with type 2 diabetes have a very high risk of heart disease because diabetes predisposes them to high blood pressure and to the buildup of fatty deposits called plaques in their arteries. This buildup of plaque is called atherosclerosis. Plaque can develop cracks at the surface and rupture, forming blood clots that can obstruct an artery. If the artery delivers blood to the heart, the blood supply to part of the heart can be cut off, blocking its supply of oxygen and nutrients and causing a heart attack. If this process occurs in the arteries that deliver blood to the brain, the result is a stroke.

For a person with type 2 diabetes, the risk of having a heart attack is 2½ times higher than normal—the same increased risk as someone without diabetes who has already had a heart attack. In addition, if you have diabetes, your chances of dying from your first heart attack are the same as that person's chances of dying from a second heart attack.

Preventing Heart Disease

In addition to controlling blood glucose, the best way for people with diabetes to avoid heart disease is to follow the heart-healthy advice recommended for everyone: eat a nutritious low-fat, high-fiber diet rich in whole grains, fruits, and vegetables; get regular exercise; and maintain a healthy weight. And treat any other health problems such as high blood pressure or abnormal blood fats (such as cholesterol and triglycerides) as soon as they are detected. For someone with prediabetes or diabetes, these measures can be lifesaving.

Control Your Blood Pressure

High blood pressure (see page 93) damages blood vessels. If you have both type 2 diabetes and high blood pressure, the damaging effect on your blood vessels is multiplied. Your blood pressure should be under 120/80. If lifestyle measures such as weight loss and exercise do not lower your blood pressure to a healthy level, your doctor will prescribe antihypertensive medication to bring it down.

Improve Your Cholesterol

You also need to get your cholesterol profile (levels of cholesterol and other lipids; see page 94) under control to reduce your risk of diabetes complications. Abnormal blood cholesterol levels are a major risk factor for heart disease. Your total cholesterol level should be below 200 mg/dL (milligrams per deciliter).

Doctors have found that a high LDL ("bad") cholesterol level is an important predictor of heart disease risk. If you already have heart disease, circulation problems, or diabetes, your LDL cholesterol should be below 100 mg/dL; some doctors recommend that people with heart risk factors get their LDL below 70. If you have two or more risk factors for heart disease—high blood pressure, smoking, a family history of heart disease, or being over age 45 (if you're a man) or over 55 (if you're a woman)—your LDL should be under 130 mg/dL. People without these risk factors or conditions should also try to keep their LDL cholesterol level below 130. The lower the LDL the better.

With HDL ("good") cholesterol, on the other hand, higher is better. Levels of 60 mg/dL or higher may help reduce the risk of heart disease, while HDL levels under 40 mg/dL increase heart disease risk.

Triglycerides are another type of blood fat to monitor if you have diabetes. Levels above 150 mg/dL are considered high. High triglyceride levels can make the cells less sensitive to insulin. Also, particles of fat that carry triglycerides absorb or take in cholesterol, lower the level of good HDL cholesterol, and slow the clearance of bad LDL cholesterol from the blood.

If you can't improve your cholesterol profile with diet, exercise, and weight loss, your doctor will probably prescribe a cholesterol-lowering medication, such as a statin (which reduces the liver's production of cholesterol).

Quit Smoking

Smoking increases the risk of heart disease on its own but it becomes especially dangerous when combined with other risk factors, such as a family history of heart disease, high blood pressure, type 2 diabetes, and high cholesterol. Cigarette smoking raises blood pressure, makes blood clot more easily, reduces stamina and tolerance for exercise, and reduces HDL (good) cholesterol. Women over 35 who take birth-control pills and smoke increase their risk of heart disease and stroke significantly. If you smoke, stop now. Ask your doctor about smoking cessation aids—such as nicotine gum, pills, and patches (sold over the counter) or nicotine inhalers and nasal sprays (available only by prescription)—and structured smoking cessation programs (such as those sponsored by the American Lung Association).

Manage Your Stress

Finding effective ways to manage stress (see page 128) can also help reduce your heart disease risk. Try relaxation techniques, deep breathing exercise, yoga, regular exercise, and meditation to keep stress in check. In addition, getting 8 hours of sleep every night can improve your ability to face life's daily challenges.

Get the Important Nutrients

Consuming at least 400 micrograms of the B vitamin folic acid every day, along with vitamins B6 and B12, reduces your levels of homocysteine, a body chemical that indicates the presence of chronic inflammation in the blood vessels. Inflammation promotes the buildup of fatty deposits in arteries that can lead to heart disease. Good sources of folic acid include green leafy vegetables; orange juice; and dried beans. Folic acid is included in daily vitamin/mineral supplements, and cereals, breads, and grains are fortified with folic acid.

Take an Aspirin a Day

Many doctors recommend a daily low dose of aspirin, such as a baby aspirin, to help prevent heart disease and stroke in people with diabetes who are over the age of 30. Aspirin has been shown to keep red blood cells from clumping together, making them less likely to form a clot that could obstruct an artery and cause a heart attack or stroke. Taking aspirin regularly can irritate the stomach lining and cause bleeding, so talk to your doctor before you start doing so. Enteric coated aspirin are less irritating to the stomach.

You can have blocked arteries and not know it because developing heart disease often produces no noticeable symptoms. For some people, the first awareness of heart disease comes when they have a heart attack. Other people have chest pain (angina) that occurs when the heart muscle temporarily receives an insufficient amount of oxygen. Angina is more likely to occur during exercise or periods of emotional stress. The pain usually stops with rest—heart attack pain, by contrast, does *not* stop with rest.

Warning Signs of a Heart Attack

A heart attack usually produces physical symptoms, but not everyone who is having a heart attack has the same symptoms, and women can have different symptoms than men. Become familiar with the signs of a heart attack so you can act immediately if they occur. Don't delay if you think you could be having a heart attack; the sooner you get treatment, the less damage to your heart and the better your outcome is likely to be. Call 911 and, while you are waiting, chew on a regular aspirin (not an enteric-coated one), which thins the blood and may help prevent damage to the heart. Do not try to drive yourself to the hospital because you could lose consciousness while driving.

Following are the most common symptoms of a heart attack:

- Crushing chest pain or tight pressure around the chest
- Pain or discomfort in the arms, back, jaw, neck, or stomach
- Shortness of breath
- Indigestion or nausea
- Breaking out in a cold sweat

Many women think they are not as likely to have a heart attack as men—but they are wrong. Heart disease is the top killer of both men and women in the United States. On average, women are about 10 years older than men when they have their first heart attack, and they often have different warning signs. Although the most common warning sign of a heart attack in women is chest pain or discomfort, as in men, women are more likely than men to experience the following symptoms:

- Shortness of breath
- Severe fatigue
- Indigestion, nausea, or vomiting
- Back, jaw, or shoulder pain
- Dizziness or light-headedness

Diagnosing Heart Disease

If you have angina, or several risk factors for heart disease, your doctor may refer you to a cardiologist (a doctor who specializes in treating heart problems). Your doctor or cardiologist will probably put you through a series of tests such as those below to diagnose heart disease.

Electrocardiogram

An electrocardiogram (ECG) measures the electrical activity of the heart muscle and allows doctors to detect any arrhythmias (abnormal heartbeats). An ECG can also spot ischemia, which is inadequate blood flow to the heart.

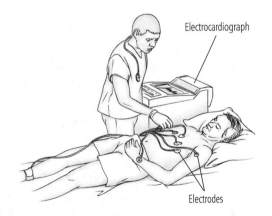

Electrocardiograph

Electrodes

Electrocardiogram

During an electrocardiogram, the doctor or a technician will place electrodes on your chest, arms, and legs to measure and record the electrical activity of your heart.

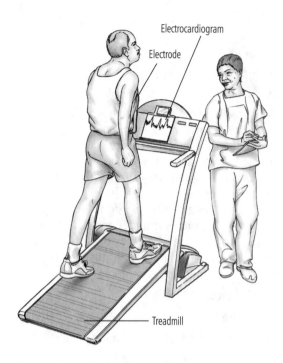

Electrocardiogram

Electrode

Treadmill

Exercise Stress Test

An exercise stress test helps doctors evaluate the severity of heart disease and reveals how well the heart responds to an insufficient blood supply.

Exercise Stress Test

For an exercise stress test, you have an ECG while you walk or run on an exercise treadmill or ride a stationary bicycle to check for abnormal heart beats or inadequate blood supply to the heart during physical exertion. A similar test, called a thallium exercise stress test, tracks the movement of a radioactive dye through the bloodstream both during exertion and while at rest.

Echocardiogram

An echocardiogram uses sound waves to produce images that show the size of the heart (diseased or damaged hearts are often enlarged), its pumping action, blood flow, and valve function. In people with inadequate blood flow to the heart, the pumping motion of the heart's left ventricle appears abnormal on an echocardiogram. A stress echocardiogram combines an exercise stress test with the echocardiogram.

Echocardiogram

During an echocardiogram, a technician places a device called a transducer on the left side of the chest over the rib cage. The transducer transmits sound waves that are converted into an image on a computer screen.

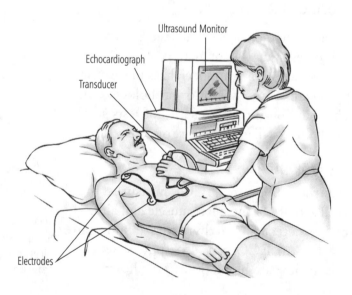

Ultrasound Monitor

Echocardiograph

Transducer

Electrodes

Coronary Angiogram

Doctors perform an angiogram, also known as cardiac catheterization, to more closely examine the inside of the arteries that lead to the heart. For this procedure, a thin, flexible tube (catheter) is inserted into a large blood vessel (usually in the groin area) and threaded up through the aorta (the body's main artery) into the arteries leading to the heart. After injecting a dye into the catheter, the doctor takes a series of rapid-sequence X-rays of the artery he or she thinks may be blocked. The X-ray images will show exactly where and how complete any blockages are.

CT Scan

A computed tomography (CT) scan takes cross-sectional X-ray images of the heart and its arteries as the patient lies on a table that slides through a ring-shaped machine. These images can detect calcium particles in the fatty deposits in the arteries leading to the heart. These calcified deposits, or plaques, are an indication of heart disease.

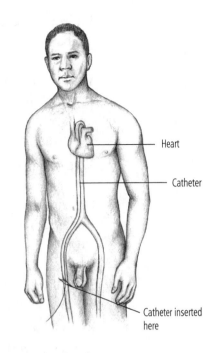

Heart

Catheter

Catheter inserted here

Coronary Angiogram

The X-rays produced during a coronary angiogram help doctors detect blockages in arteries leading to the heart. The images can help them determine how to treat the blockages.

Cardiac MRI

Magnetic resonance imaging (MRI) uses radiofrequency waves and a strong magnetic field instead of X-rays to provide images of internal organs and tissues. The images are taken as the person lies on a table that slides through a ring-shaped machine. Cardiac MRI enables doctors to examine the structures of the heart and major blood vessels, evaluate their function, and detect damage to the heart from a heart attack or heart disease.

Treating Heart Disease

Scientists have developed a multitude of different medications—including beta blockers, ACE inhibitors, diuretics, digitalis preparations, and anticoagulants—to treat heart disease. After a thorough examination, your doctor will decide which medication will best improve blood flow to your heart and relieve your chest pain. You will probably have to take this medication for the rest of your life.

Doctors perform a number of procedures that can redirect blood vessels around a blocked artery or reopen an obstructed artery, including the following.

Coronary Artery Bypass Surgery

Bypass surgery is widely used to treat the buildup of fatty deposits in an artery by grafting healthy blood vessels from other parts of the body (usually the leg) onto the affected artery to reroute blood flow around the blockage. Most grafted arteries stay open for at least 10 years after surgery.

Balloon Angioplasty

To open a blocked artery in people who have chronic angina (chest pain), doctors use a procedure called angioplasty in which a tube (catheter) with a balloon at its tip is inserted into the affected artery. The doctor then inflates the balloon to press the fatty deposits (plaques) against the wall of the artery. A metallic or plastic wire mesh called a stent is often placed at the site to keep the artery open and reduce the risk of reblockage. Some stents slowly release medication that helps prevent the overgrowth of scar tissue that can lead to reblockage.

Radiation Therapy

Radiation therapy (called vascular brachytherapy) is sometimes used in addition to stent placement if an artery has become reblocked after angioplasty. Low-dose radiation (in the form of tiny radioactive pellets inserted through a catheter into the area of the blockage) is given for about 5 minutes after stent placement to prevent scar tissue from forming around the stent.

Other Artery-Opening Procedures

In a procedure called atherectomy, doctors thread a tiny instrument through a catheter into a blocked artery to shave the plaque away in very thin layers. The shavings are then removed through the catheter. In a procedure called laser angioplasty, doctors use a highly concentrated beam of light (laser) to vaporize the blockage.

Stroke

Your brain needs a steady supply of oxygen and nutrients to keep working properly, and it relies on a system of blood vessels to deliver them. When a vessel becomes blocked, blood can't reach part of the brain. After 3 or 4 minutes, that part of the brain begins to lose its ability to function. A stroke occurs when the blood supply to part of the brain is cut off by a blockage in an artery or, less often, by a ruptured artery in the brain. A stroke damages brain tissue, usually causing some type of reduced function, such as paralysis or speech impairment, depending on the area of the brain affected. The impairment may be temporary or permanent.

Diabetes and Stroke Risk

Having type 2 diabetes or even prediabetes places you at a much higher risk of having a stroke than people without diabetes—even if all other risk factors are equal. As with heart attack, the risk of stroke is 2½ times

---

WARNING!

The Warning Signs of a Stroke

A stroke is a medical emergency. If you think you or someone you are with may be having a stroke, call 911 immediately so you can get potentially lifesaving medical treatment quickly. The warning signs of a stroke often first become noticeable in the morning, just after a person wakes up. Following are the most common signs of an impending stroke:

- Sudden, intense headache
- Numbness or weakness in the face, arm, or leg, usually on one side of the body
- A weak grip
- Sudden nausea and vomiting
- Slurred speech
- Difficulty understanding spoken words
- Blurred or reduced vision in one or both eyes
- Difficulty swallowing
- Poor balance, clumsiness, or difficulty walking
- Inability to read or understand

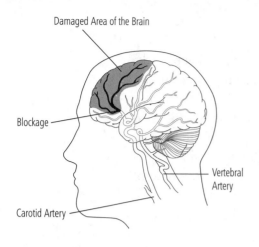

Damaged Area of the Brain

Blockage

Vertebral Artery

Carotid Artery

Blocked Artery in the Brain

A stroke occurs when a blood vessel in the brain becomes blocked, cutting off the blood supply to that part of the brain. Blockage of blood flow to one side of the brain usually produces symptoms (such as numbness or paralysis) on the opposite side of the body.

higher than normal for both men and women with type 2 diabetes. When people with diabetes have a stroke, their outlook for survival and complete recovery is often poorer than that of people who don't have diabetes. The reason for this disparity is that people with diabetes often have circulation problems, high blood pressure, and abnormal blood fats, which have an effect on blood vessels as well as on a person's overall health. Obesity and inactivity also play a role in a person's ability to recover from a stroke.

Treating Stroke

Doctors can treat most strokes (except for those caused by ruptured blood vessels and bleeding in the brain) with a clot-busting medication called tPA (tissue plasminogen activator), which dissolves the blood clot that is blocking the artery, allowing blood flow to the brain to resume. To be successful, tPA must be given within the first 3 hours after stroke symptoms appear—which is why getting to the hospital quickly is so important. Sometimes doctors treat stroke with surgery that removes the plaque from inside the affected artery or with angioplasty (in which a balloon is inserted into the artery and inflated to open the blockage) or another artery-opening procedure (see page 172).

Preventing Stroke

Having high blood pressure (see page 93) is the number one risk factor for stroke. Having elevated LDL (bad) cholesterol and diabetes also increase stroke risk. That's why it is so important to have your blood pressure, cholesterol levels, and blood glucose levels checked by your doctor on a regular basis. If you have high blood pressure, your doctor will prescribe medication to lower it. A group of medications called ACE inhibitors is frequently used to treat high blood pressure in people who have diabetes because these medications also prevent or delay the development of kidney disease, which can be a complication of diabetes.

The Stroke Test

Here is a quick technique developed by researchers at the University of Cincinnati to enable paramedics to quickly determine if someone may have had a stroke. Officially called the Cincinnati Prehospital Stroke Scale but popularly referred to as the Talk, Wave, Smile Test, it describes how to rapidly check three physical findings that are telltale signs of stroke: one-sided facial droop, inability to raise one arm, and difficulty with speech. The test is so easy that even children can perform it. Follow these three simple steps quickly if you suspect someone has had a stroke, and if the person cannot do any one of them, call 911 or your local emergency number immediately.

1. Ask the person to smile.
   - Normal response: Both sides of the face move equally.
   - Abnormal response: One side of the face does not move (looks like it's drooping).

2. Ask the person to close his or her eyes and hold both arms out straight for 10 seconds.
   - Normal response: Both arms move equally or are held at a steady position.
   - Abnormal response: One arm cannot move or drifts down.

3. Ask the person to say "Don't cry over spilled milk."
   - Normal response: The person says the correct words with no slurring.
   - Abnormal response: The person slurs the words, says the wrong words, or can't speak at all.

In addition to an ACE inhibitor, your doctor may also prescribe other medications such as diuretics (which help the body remove excess water and sodium) and beta blockers (which block the heartbeat-increasing effects of the stress hormone adrenaline). Beta blockers regulate the heartbeat and lower the heart's need for blood and oxygen by reducing its workload. Calcium channel blockers, another class of blood pressure medication, cause blood vessels to relax by blocking their intake of calcium.

Changes in your diet and increased physical activity can reduce atherosclerosis (the buildup of fatty deposits inside artery walls). Another major step you can take to prevent stroke is to stop smoking if you smoke. Cigarette smoking is one of the most important risk factors for heart disease and stroke, and smoking can make the cells resistant to insulin, making it harder to control blood glucose.

Circulation Problems

The same blood vessel blockages from fatty deposits that cause heart attack and stroke can affect the blood vessels in the legs, causing diminished blood flow to the legs and feet. About one in every three people over age 50 who has type 2 diabetes has this circulation disorder, known medically as peripheral artery disease, to some degree. Having circulation problems also indicates a high risk of heart disease, heart attack, and stroke.

Many people with peripheral artery disease have no symptoms and do not know they have circulation problems. Others may have mild leg pain or difficulty walking that they attribute to aging. When symptoms occur, you may experience the following:

- Leg pain when walking or exercising that goes away with rest
- Numbness and tingling in the lower legs and feet
- Cold legs and feet
- Wounds or infections on the feet and legs that take a long time to heal

To diagnose circulation problems, your doctor will probably measure the blood pressure in your ankle and compare it with the blood pressure in your arm. Having a lower blood pressure reading in the lower leg than in the arm is a strong sign of circulation problems. To confirm the diagnosis, the doctor may also order an angiogram (see page 171), which uses X-rays to detect blockages in arteries after dye has been injected into them; an ultrasound, which uses sound waves to construct images to identify blocked arteries; or an MRI (magnetic resonance imaging), which uses magnetic waves to detect blood vessel obstructions.

People who have circulation problems are at very high risk of developing heart disease and of having a heart attack or stroke. If you have circulation problems, you should be especially diligent about controlling your blood glucose, keeping your blood pressure under 120/80 mm Hg, and bringing your LDL (bad) cholesterol down below 100 mg/dL, perhaps even to 70 mg/dL if your doctor recommends. Walking an hour every day is an excellent way to keep your blood flowing.

In severe cases, doctors treat circulation problems with a procedure called angioplasty (see page 172), in which a tiny tube attached to a balloon is inserted into a blocked artery; once inside, the balloon is inflated to widen the artery. A metal or plastic wire mesh called a stent is then sometimes inserted into the blocked area to keep the artery open. An alternative procedure is an artery bypass graft, which uses a healthy blood vessel taken from another part of the body to reroute blood flow around the blocked artery.

Cigarette smoking contributes to circulation problems in two main ways. When you inhale cigarette smoke, nicotine (the addictive chemical in tobacco) triggers a rush of adrenaline that causes stored fat to be released into the bloodstream. The carbon monoxide present in the smoke damages the delicate layer of cells that lines the inner walls of blood vessels, making it easier for fatty deposits to stick to the blood vessel walls. If you smoke, this double threat occurs in every blood vessel in your body, increasing your risk of having a heart attack or a stroke.

Nerve Damage

Damage to the nerves that connect the spinal cord to muscles, blood vessels, skin, and internal organs is one of the most common chronic complications of type 2 diabetes. Doctors call this peripheral neuropathy because it affects primarily the peripheral nerves, those that carry messages between the central nervous system (the brain and the spinal cord) and the rest of the body. However, peripheral neuropathy can also affect the nerves that control automatic functions such as breathing and heartbeat.

There are three main types of peripheral nerves: motor, sensory, and autonomic. Motor nerves transmit signals to the muscles to initiate movements such as lifting an arm or walking. Sensory nerves carry impulses in the opposite direction—from the senses (sight, hearing, touch, smell, taste, and balance) to the brain. Sensory nerves also convey pain messages to the brain. Autonomic nerves transmit messages to the brain about body functions over which you have no control, such as breathing, heartbeat, digestion, and the release of hormones. Elevated levels of glucose in the blood can cause damage to any of these nerves.

Nerve damage from diabetes can be painful and disabling. The most common symptoms of nerve damage include numbness, a tingling or prickly sensation, and burning pain, usually in the feet and legs but sometimes also in the hands. The feet can become so painful that walking or standing becomes difficult. Nerve damage can affect only one side of the body but usually affects both sides. These symptoms result from the increased activity of nerves when they are damaged or are in the process of healing.

People with nerve damage often lose the ability to feel in the affected area. Loss of feeling in the foot, for example, can lead to an inability to feel the position of the foot, causing the ankle joint to become unstable. Your foot can become injured and, because you can't feel the pain, you don't realize your foot is injured. An ingrown toenail or a small wound on the foot can go unnoticed until infection sets in. If surrounding blood vessels are also damaged, the wound may not heal and can become a chronic foot ulcer. Eventually, the tissue can die (gangrene) and amputation of the affected area may be necessary. Nerve damage in people with diabetes is the most common cause of amputation in the United States.

Nerve damage can have other harmful effects as well, including muscle weakness, erection problems (see page 190), diarrhea, constipation, and recurring urinary tract infections.

To diagnose peripheral neuropathy, your doctor will ask you to describe your pain and other symptoms. He or she may also perform tests to evaluate your muscle strength and sensation by, for example, observing whether you can feel a vibration or a prick with a dull pin. Some tests use mild electric shocks to measure the speed with which impulses travel along a nerve.

In some cases, nerve damage lasts only a few months and goes away on its own, but in most cases the condition is chronic and gets worse. Because doctors do not yet know how to heal nerves damaged by type 2 diabetes, treatment seeks mainly to improve the symptoms. To relieve pain, doctors often recommend over-the-counter pain remedies such as ibuprofen. Prescription medications such as imipramine (an antidepressant) and gabapentin (used to treat seizures in epilepsy) have been shown to relieve pain from diabetic nerve damage. Capsaicin creams, which contain extracts of hot chili peppers, can be applied to the skin to help obstruct pain signals. Pain relievers work best if you use them regularly over the course of the day, before the pain becomes severe. Prescription narcotic drugs relieve pain, but doctors use them cautiously because of the risk of addiction.

Doctors do not yet understand precisely how diabetes causes nerve damage, but blood sugar control seems to play a key role in preventing it because nerve damage is worse in people who have had diabetes for a long time and in those who have difficulty controlling their blood sugar. Not smoking and avoiding excessive alcohol intake can also help reduce your risk of having nerve damage. Reaching and staying at a healthy weight and engaging in regular physical activity can help prevent any nerve damage from worsening.

Daily Foot Checks

High blood sugar levels from diabetes can cause two problems that can harm your feet: nerve damage and poor blood flow. Having damaged nerves makes you less likely to feel pain, heat, or cold in your legs and feet. Because you don't feel pain, you may not realize you have a sore or a cut on your foot and it could get larger or become infected. Poor blood circulation reduces blood flow to your legs and feet, making it harder for a foot sore or infection to heal. If you smoke, these blood flow problems can be even worse.

Together, nerve damage and poor circulation can result in severe foot ulcers. In extreme cases, infected foot ulcers never heal and the skin and tissue around the sore begin to die, turning black. This condition is called gangrene. To keep gangrene from spreading up the leg, a surgeon may have to amputate the affected toe, foot, or part of the leg.

Even such common foot problems as corns and calluses can cause serious problems for a person with diabetes. Other common foot ailments that can lead to infections in people with diabetes include ingrown toenails, blisters, bunions, plantar warts, hammertoes, and athlete's foot—even dry cracked skin can be a problem. Watch for these foot problems and, if you notice any, bring them to your doctor's attention right away.

The most important thing you can do to take care of your feet is to check them every day for anything unusual. Set a specific time each day to do it so it becomes a habit and you won't forget. If you can't bend over to see your feet, use a mirror. If you can't see very well, ask someone else to check your feet for you. Ask your doctor to recommend a podiatrist (foot doctor) who can cut your toenails if you can't do it yourself. Here are some other tips to help you keep your feet healthy:

- Wash your feet in lukewarm water every day. Test the water temperature with your elbow, not your foot. Dry your feet thoroughly, especially between the toes.

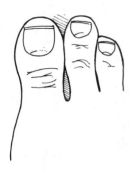

- If your skin is dry, rub lotion on your feet after you wash and dry them.
- File corns and calluses gently with an emery board or a pumice stone after you bathe; don't use a razor blade or a knife.
  - Cut your toenails once a week. Cut them when they are soft, after bathing. Cut them straight across, but not too short, and file them with an emery board. Do not cut into the corners of the toes.
  - Always wear shoes or slippers to protect your feet.
  - Wear socks or stockings to prevent blisters. Don't wear knee-high nylon stockings because they can get too tight below the knee and reduce blood flow even more.
- Make sure your shoes fit properly. Shop for shoes at the end of the day when your feet are largest. Break in new shoes slowly—wear them for 1 or 2 hours a day for the first couple of weeks.
- Before you put on your shoes, check to make sure nothing sharp (such as a pebble) has fallen into them.
- Keep the blood flowing to your feet. Put your feet up, wiggle your toes, and move your feet up and down from the ankle a few times each day.
- Ask your doctor to examine your feet at least once a year.

Foot ulcers most often appear on the ball of the foot or on the bottom of the big toe. Poorly fitting shoes are a common cause of ulcers on the sides of the feet. See your doctor right away if you notice any sores or broken skin areas while you are checking your feet because ignoring a sore can lead to infection, and infection is the leading cause of limb loss from amputation.

Skin Problems

Diabetes affects every part of the body, including the skin. Up to a third of all people with type 2 diabetes have skin problems from the disease. In fact, for some people, a skin disorder is the first noticeable sign of diabetes. People with type 2 diabetes are more likely than people without the disorder to develop certain skin conditions, and some skin conditions occur exclusively in people with diabetes.

Type 2 diabetes can affect your skin in two ways. First, when your blood sugar is high, your body loses fluid, which can make the skin dry. Second, nerve damage from diabetes can inhibit sweating (sweating helps keep the skin soft and moist). Scratching itchy, dry skin can cause it to become sore, providing a site for germs to enter and cause infection. Below are some common skin problems experienced by people with type 2 diabetes.

Bacterial Infections

Common infections caused by bacteria that affect people with diabetes include sties (infections of the glands in the eyelid), infections of the hair follicles, carbuncles (deep skin infections), and infections around the fingernails and toenails. Doctors treat bacterial infections with antibiotics.

Fungal Infections

People with diabetes are especially susceptible to infection with the fungus *Candida albicans*, a type of yeast. Yeast infections usually develop in warm folds of the skin, such as under the breasts, between the fingers and toes, in the corners of the mouth, in the armpits, and in the groin. Fungal infections produce itchy, red areas surrounded by blisters and scales. Yeast infections can also occur in the mouth, where they are referred to as thrush. Jock itch, athlete's foot, ringworm, and vaginal yeast infections are also common fungal infections. Prescription antifungal creams are used to treat these infections.

Acanthosis Nigricans

Usually found in people who are obese, especially children and young adults, acanthosis nigricans (see page 207) is characterized by slightly raised, brown patches on the neck, armpits, and groin. Losing weight can help make the patches disappear.

Necrobiosis Lipoidica Diabeticorum

While it affects only 1 out of 300 people with diabetes, this rare leg disorder can be disfiguring. It produces round, large, slightly indented red or purple patches of skin that can be painful and sometimes crack open. Women are three times more likely than men to have this disorder.

Diabetic Dermopathy

Diabetic dermopathy is characterized by round, light brown, scaly patches, especially on the shins. This condition arises from changes in the small blood vessels of the skin caused by diabetes. The disorder is harmless and needs no treatment.

Keeping Your Skin Healthy

If you have diabetes, taking good care of your skin can help reduce your risk of serious skin problems. Here are some general guidelines for keeping your skin healthy:

- Keep your blood glucose under good control. High blood sugar can make the skin dry and can reduce the immune system's ability to fight harmful bacteria, increasing the risk of skin infections.
- Keep your skin clean and dry. Wash with a mild soap and rinse and dry your skin well, especially in skin folds under the arms and breasts and between the fingers and toes.
- Avoid very hot baths and showers. If your skin is dry, avoid bubble baths and use only mild, moisturizing soaps and mild shampoos. Do *not* use feminine hygiene sprays.
- After bathing, use an oil-in-water skin cream that doesn't contain alcohol; ask your doctor to recommend a lotion. (Don't put lotion between your toes because the extra moisture there can encourage the growth of fungus.)
- Never scratch. Scratching dry or itchy skin can produce open sores that attract germs.
- Wear all-cotton underwear, which allows air to move around your body.
- Check your skin regularly for dry, red, or sore spots that could become infected. Treat cuts right away: wash minor cuts with soap and water and cover them with sterile gauze. Do *not* use an antiseptic, alcohol, or iodine to clean a cut because these products are too harsh; use an antibiotic cream or ointment *only* if your doctor says it's okay to do so. See your doctor right away if you have a major cut, burn, or infection.
- During cold, dry months, keep your home more humid and try to bathe less frequently.
- See a dermatologist (a doctor who specializes in skin disorders) about any skin problems you are not able to clear up quickly yourself.

Eye Damage

Diabetes can damage the eyes in a number of ways. The three most common eye problems associated with diabetes are diabetic retinopathy, glaucoma, and cataracts. Because these complications can often be slowed or corrected with early treatment, it's essential to have your eyes examined at least once a year by an eye doctor (ophthalmologist). Of course, it is best to take steps to avoid eye damage before it occurs, and the most effective way to prevent eye problems is to keep your blood sugar levels as close to normal as possible. Minimizing exposure to the sun and not smoking may also help reduce your risk of cataracts.

Diabetic Retinopathy

Diabetic retinopathy is the most common diabetes-induced eye problem. Retinopathy results from damage to the tiny blood vessels inside the retina (the light-sensitive membrane that lines the back of the eye). The condition usually affects both eyes. In industrialized countries, diabetic retinopathy is the chief cause of irreversible blindness. If you have diabetic retinopathy, you may not at first notice any changes to your vision but, over time, as the blood vessel damage worsens, you will begin to experience loss of vision.

Diabetic retinopathy occurs in four stages. During the first stage, tiny areas of balloonlike swelling develop in the blood vessels of the retina. In stage two, blood vessels that nourish the retina become obstructed. As more blood vessels become blocked, in stage three, new blood vessels begin to grow to compensate for the damaged ones. In the final stage, these new blood vessels proliferate rapidly, but they are abnormal and fragile. If they begin to leak blood, they can cause severe vision loss—even blindness. During any stage of diabetic retinopathy, fluid can leak into the macula (the part of the retina responsible for sharp, central vision), causing the retina to swell and producing blind spots in the center of the visual field.

If you have early symptoms of diabetic retinopathy, you will see a few specks of blood or spots that appear to be floating in your central vision. They may clear up without treatment but frequently recur, causing reduced vision. Diabetic retinopathy often has no early warning signs. However, because it can progress to blindness if not treated, do not wait for symptoms to appear. If you have diabetes, it's especially

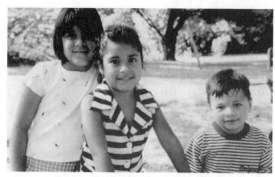
Normal Vision

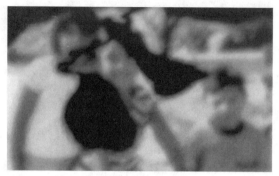
Vision Affected by Diabetic Retinopathy

Vision Loss from Diabetic Retinopathy

Diabetic retinopathy damages the retina, the light-sensitive membrane that lines the back of the eye. Vision becomes blurred and blind spots appear in the center of your field of vision. Over time, diabetic retinopathy can cause permanent vision loss or total blindness.

important to have a comprehensive eye exam at least once a year to uncover any hidden problems and get them treated at an early stage, when treatment is most effective.

Treating Diabetic Retinopathy

Doctors treat diabetic retinopathy with laser surgery (which uses high-energy light beams) to shrink the abnormal blood vessels that are growing in the retina. Laser treatment is most effective when performed before the fragile, new blood vessels have begun to bleed. If bleeding inside the retina is already severe, you may need to have a surgical procedure called a vitrectomy, during which the surgeon removes blood from the center of the eye.

Swelling of the retina is also treated with laser surgery. The laser bursts seal the bleeding blood vessels to slow the leaking of fluid and reduce the overall amount of fluid in the retina. This type of laser surgery can lower the risk of vision loss by up to 50 percent.

Glaucoma

In glaucoma, pressure from an increase in undrained fluid builds up inside the eye, causing damage to the optic nerve (the nerve that sends visual signals to the brain). Glaucoma causes gradual loss of peripheral (side) vision, resulting in narrow, tunnel-like vision that can, if untreated, eventually progress to complete blindness. Although glaucoma has a strong inherited factor, it affects people who have diabetes 40 percent more often than it does the general population.

Treating Glaucoma

Damage to the optic nerve from glaucoma is usually permanent, but treatment can slow the disease or prevent it from getting worse. Eye doctors treat glaucoma by prescribing eye drops that lower the pressure in the eye. You will have to take the drops for the rest of your life to control the pressure. If the eye drops fail to work or if you have an allergic reaction to them, laser surgery can be done to permanently alter the angle of drainage and allow fluid to more easily drain away from the eye. The laser surgery for glaucoma is painless.

Cataracts

A cataract is a clouding of the lens of the eye from a buildup of protein fibers that causes blurred or distorted vision. People with diabetes have a 60 percent higher risk of developing cataracts than people without diabetes, and they get them at an earlier age.

Treating Cataracts

To treat cataracts, doctors surgically remove the clouded lens of a mature cataract and insert a new replacement lens. Cataract surgery, which has a 98 percent success rate in restoring vision, takes an hour or less, you go home the same day, and you'll probably be able to resume your usual activities within a few days.

Have Regular Eye Exams

If you have type 2 diabetes, you should see an ophthalmologist (a doctor who specializes in diseases of the eye) at least once a year. If you already have diabetic retinopathy, you may need to have your eyes examined more often than once a year. An ophthalmologist can check for diabetic retinopathy and glaucoma using a series of tests.

A visual acuity test measures how well you can see at various distances. The visual field test evaluates your peripheral vision. For a dilated eye exam, the doctor places drops in your eyes that widen or dilate the pupils to enable him or her to see (through a magnifying lens) any damage to the optic nerve or the retina. In the dilated eye exam, the doctor can spot early signs of diabetic retinopathy, including leaking blood vessels, swelling of the retina, and damaged nerve tissue. An eye exam called tonometry measures the pressure inside the eye, which helps diagnose glaucoma.

Kidney Disease

The kidneys contain millions of microscopic blood vessels that filter out waste products from the blood. Diabetes can damage these tiny blood vessels in the same way that it damages the blood vessels in other parts of the body. High levels of blood sugar force the kidneys to filter too much blood. Over time, the kidneys become overworked and start to leak. Proteins that normally circulate in the blood spill into the urine. At a later stage, waste products begin to accumulate in the blood. Eventually, the kidneys may no longer be able to remove the waste products and they begin to fail.

Because the kidneys are good at compensating for their failing blood vessels, kidney disease produces no symptoms until function is almost completely gone. Initial symptoms of kidney failure include fluid buildup in the tissues, loss of appetite, sleep loss, nausea and vomiting, weakness, and difficulty concentrating. Eventually, urination decreases, sometimes to less than a cup of urine a day. You may have persistent swelling in the legs and feet. Without treatment, kidney failure produces drowsiness, confusion, seizures, coma, and eventually death.

Only 10 to 20 percent of all people with diabetes develop kidney disease. Still, the possibility of kidney disease is another strong incentive to see your doctor on a regular basis. During a routine checkup, your doctor can take your blood pressure (high blood pressure can cause kidney disease) and order a special urine test to check for the presence of a specific protein (microalbumin) in your urine, which can be a sign of kidney disease.

Like other potential complications of diabetes, kidney disease can be prevented by keeping blood sugar under control. Maintaining a normal blood pressure is also important because a small rise in blood pressure can rapidly make kidney disease worse. If you can't control your blood pressure with diet, weight control, and exercise, your doctor may prescribe blood pressure medication. Medications called ACE inhibitors are especially good for people who have high blood pressure and kidney disease because they slow the progression of kidney disease. To monitor the health of your kidneys, your doctor will recommend regular kidney function tests.

Treating Kidney Disease

If you have advanced kidney disease, your doctor may put you on a low-protein diet because consuming too much protein can make your already overtaxed kidneys work even harder. The normal daily requirement for protein is surprisingly small—only 0.8 gram of protein per kilogram (2.2 pounds) of body weight. To lower your protein intake, your doctor may recommend limiting protein to 0.6 gram per kilogram of body weight.

If your kidneys fail, you will need to have kidney dialysis, a treatment in which a machine takes over the function of the kidneys on a regular basis. If your kidney failure is permanent, you will need dialysis for the rest of your life. There are two types of dialysis—hemodialysis and peritoneal dialysis. During hemodialysis, your blood flows through a tube into a machine called a dialysis unit. The dialysis unit filters impurities out of the blood and sends it back into your body through another tube. A dialysis treatment usually lasts about 4 hours and is repeated two or three times a week, depending on the degree of kidney failure.

Peritoneal dialysis is done without a machine. The doctor makes a small incision in the abdomen, inserts a thin plastic tube, and infuses a special solution into the abdomen that absorbs waste products from the blood. After several hours, the waste-containing fluid drains out of the abdomen. Many people learn how to perform daily peritoneal dialysis themselves, at home. Both types of dialysis can have side effects, such as anemia, bone disease, and nutrient deficiencies. Good control of blood sugar remains important during kidney dialysis.

For some people with kidney failure, a kidney transplant is the best option for survival. The waiting period to acquire a new kidney is long because donor organs are in short supply, but the body can function normally with just one working kidney. After a kidney transplant, you must take medications that suppress your immune system because otherwise your body would recognize the new kidney as foreign and reject it. Keep in mind that having a new kidney will not cure your diabetes and, without strict control of your blood sugar, diabetes can eventually damage the transplanted kidney as well.

Gum Disease

Diabetes and gum disease (also known as periodontal disease) have a complex two-way relationship. People with type 2 diabetes—especially those whose blood sugar levels are poorly controlled—have a much higher than normal risk of developing gum disease. Gum infections take longer to heal and, if they become chronic, can lead to tooth loss. Conversely, having gum disease can make your diabetes worse by making your blood sugar harder to control.

Gum disease is a serious bacterial infection that destroys the fibers and bone that hold the teeth in the mouth. Eventually, the gums separate from the teeth, forming pockets that fill with plaque (a colorless layer of bacteria that sticks to the teeth, especially near the gums). As these pockets become more and more infected, more gum tissue and bone are destroyed and the teeth can become loose. In the United States, about 15 percent of young adults and 30 percent of people over the age of 50 have periodontal disease.

Gum disease is even more prevalent and more severe in people with type 2 diabetes and causes greater tooth loss than in the general population. The blood vessel damage that occurs from diabetes makes the gums more vulnerable to infection that can break down the gums and the bones that hold the teeth in the jaw. People with diabetes also have high amounts of sugar in their saliva, which can encourage the growth of infection-causing bacteria. The risk of both diabetes and gum disease grows higher with age. However, more and more obese adolescents and young adults are developing both type 2 diabetes and gum disease.

The first stage of periodontal disease is called gingivitis. Do your gums bleed when you brush your teeth? This bleeding is one of the first signs of gingivitis. Bacteria colonize the margin of the gums, causing the gums to become inflamed, which makes them red and swollen. The body mounts an immune response to fight the bacteria, but the inflammatory immune response itself, combined with the damage caused by

Keeping Your Teeth and Gums Healthy

Treatment for gum disease is essential, but prevention is even more important. The most effective way to prevent gum disease is to control your blood sugar. Taking good care of your teeth and gums is also important. Brush your teeth with a soft-bristled brush at least twice a day and floss your teeth every day. If you notice that your gums bleed when you brush your teeth, see your dentist right away. Have a dental checkup and professional cleaning every six months or as often as your dentist recommends. Be sure to tell your dentist that you have diabetes and ask him or her to show you the best way to maintain healthy teeth and gums at home.

the bacteria, destroys connective tissue fibers and creates pockets around the teeth in which still more bacteria can multiply. If gingivitis progresses to mild periodontal disease, a dentist can detect receding gums and evidence of bone erosion around the tooth on an X-ray. During advanced (stage three) periodontal disease, a person can have loose teeth, bad breath, pus between the teeth and gums, and altered jaw alignment. If you have dentures, they may not fit properly because the bone surrounding your teeth has become damaged. In addition, wearing dentures can promote the growth of a yeast called *Candida albicans*, which causes oral thrush, a mouth infection common in people with diabetes.

Infected gums can make your diabetes worse by making it harder to control your blood sugar because infection in any part of the body causes blood sugar to rise. Severe gum disease can also make chewing painful, steering you toward soft foods, such as cooked noodles or mashed potatoes, which are easy to chew but may not be part of your recommended meal plan, especially in large quantities. The same delayed wound healing characteristic of type 2 diabetes that causes foot ulcers to develop also delays the healing of infected gums.

There is a link between gum disease and heart disease, and people with type 2 diabetes already have a higher than normal risk of heart disease. The bacteria in diseased gums release high levels of substances into the bloodstream that trigger inflammation in other parts of the body. Inflammation plays a powerful role in the development of heart disease and reduces your ability to control your blood glucose. The bacterial components from gum disease that travel in the bloodstream may cause the liver to produce C-reactive proteins (proteins in the blood that are a sign of inflammation in the arteries and indicate heart disease risk).

If you have gum disease, your dentist will defer treatment until your blood sugar is under reasonable control, unless the infection is very severe. Treatment will begin with a thorough deep cleaning to remove dental plaque, tartar, and infected tissue. Antibiotics may also be administered in the form of a mouth rinse or a dissolving chip that is

Smoking and Gum Disease

Smoking and gum disease are an especially bad combination. Tobacco use is a major cause of gum disease because it increases the buildup of tartar (hardened plaque) on the teeth, produces deeper pockets between the teeth and gums, and quickens the loss of bone and tissue that support the teeth—all of which speed tooth loss. In fact, more than 40 percent of daily smokers over age 65 have lost teeth, compared with only 20 percent of nonsmokers. Smoking also delays healing after any kind of oral surgery or other treatment. Smokeless tobacco and regular cigar and pipe smoking can also have these effects on the gums—another good reason to give up tobacco now.

placed inside infected pockets in the gums. When gum disease is advanced, oral surgery may have to be performed to reshape or replace lost tissue.

Type 2 diabetes can affect the mouth in other ways, too. For example, having persistent dryness in the mouth is a common symptom of undetected diabetes. Mouth dryness can promote infection and tooth decay by allowing bacteria to multiply. Diabetic symptoms can also include mouth stickiness, dry lips, a burning sensation in the mouth, and mouth sores. Dry mouth can make chewing and swallowing difficult. If your mouth is dry, ask your dentist about ways to relieve this problem.

Erection Problems

Within 10 years of developing diabetes, more than 50 percent of men experience erection problems (often called erectile dysfunction or impotence), defined as the inability to achieve and maintain an erection adequate for sexual intercourse. Erection problems can also be an early sign of diabetes. By age 70, 95 percent of men who have diabetes develop erection problems.

Having an erection requires undamaged nerves and good blood flow. To produce an erection, a man's brain has to send impulses along the nerves instructing the chambers of the penis to relax to allow blood to flow in to expand and harden the penis. Nerve damage and poor circulation are two of the most common complications of type 2 diabetes. If you are having erection problems, your doctor may examine you to determine if your penis has become insensitive to touch, which would indicate nerve damage. Blood vessel damage that can lead to a heart attack or a stroke can affect the small blood vessels in the penis, causing diminished blood flow necessary to produce an erection.

High blood pressure affects most people with type 2 diabetes and some blood pressure medications can contribute to erection problems. If you are taking medication to control your blood pressure, ask your doctor if it could be the cause of your erection problems. The doctor may be able to lower the dose of the medication or prescribe a different one to see if your ability to have an erection improves.

Several treatment options are available for erection problems caused by diabetes. Medications taken by mouth (such as sildenafil, vardenafil, and tadalafil) relax the smooth muscles of the penis, allowing blood to flow in more easily. However, you cannot use these drugs if you are taking heart medications such as nitroglycerin or alpha blockers because the combination can cause dangerously low blood pressure.

Injectable erection drugs are injected directly into the penis with a tiny needle to relax the smooth muscle and widen the main artery that supplies blood to the penis, increasing blood flow to the penis to produce an erection. Urethral suppositories, which are inserted about an inch into the urethral opening in the penis, have a similar effect. Vacuum devices produce erections by pulling blood into the penis and trapping it. Inflatable penile implants are mechanical devices that are surgically implanted in the penis, scrotum, and lower abdomen; when the pump inside the scrotum is squeezed, cylinders implanted in the penis fill with fluid from a pouch implanted in the abdomen.

As with the other common chronic complications of type 2 diabetes, the most effective way to avoid erection problems is to keep your blood sugar levels as close to normal as possible.

PART FIVE

Diabetes in Children

14

Type 2 Diabetes in Children

In the past, when diabetes struck during childhood, it was almost always type 1 diabetes, which was usually referred to as juvenile diabetes. But over the past 10 years, doctors have been diagnosing type 2 diabetes (formerly known as adult-onset diabetes) in children and adolescents with alarming frequency. In fact, type 2 diabetes is becoming one of the most common chronic diseases in children and adolescents. In the United States, more than 39,000 adolescents have type 2 diabetes and nearly 3 million have elevated fasting glucose levels. Doctors expect the numbers to continue to rise. The disorder is most likely to develop between ages 10 and 19.

The longer a person has type 2 diabetes, the greater his or her risk of complications. Over time, high blood sugar levels—and the high blood pressure and blood fat abnormalities that often accompany them—can damage cells, tissues, and organs. This damage can eventually lead to nerve problems, kidney failure, blood vessel damage, and blindness. Doctors are already seeing diabetes complications in some adolescents who have type 2 diabetes, including early onset of heart disease. If their diabetes goes uncontrolled, these young people are at increased risk of disability and early death.

The Increase in Type 2 Diabetes in Children

Until the mid-1980s, doctors defined type 2 diabetes as a condition of the middle-aged and elderly, usually acquired after years of being overweight from poor eating habits and lack of exercise. Now, it appears that these same factors are producing type 2 diabetes in adolescents and children as young as 5. While type 1 diabetes remains the most common form of the disease in children, experts predict that type 2 diabetes could become the predominant form in the next few decades. The number of children and adolescents with type 2 diabetes has increased 15-fold in the past generation and tripled in the past decade. Because the disorder may not produce symptoms early in its course, many cases in children probably remain undiagnosed for varying lengths of time.

In children, as in adults, type 2 diabetes is more strongly linked with being overweight than with any other condition. More than 90 percent of children diagnosed with type 2 diabetes in the United States are obese. The increasing weight and decreasing level of physical activity among young people are major causes of the increase in type 2 diabetes among children and young adults. When they are first diagnosed with type 2 diabetes, children and adolescents are generally between 10 and 19 years old, are significantly overweight, have a strong family history of type 2 diabetes, and have insulin resistance (a condition in which their cells don't respond properly to the hormone insulin; see page 12).

For many American children, everyday life can conspire to raise their risk of type 2 diabetes. Many are sedentary—they aren't walking to school or playing outside with friends as much as children used to. Much of the blame can be placed on the increase in sedentary activities such as watching TV and playing video games. But safety is also a concern; many parents hesitate to allow their young children to leave the house, or even play in the backyard, without adult supervision. In some communities, sidewalks can be unsafe for walking and parks unsafe for playing.

In their struggle to improve academic performance, many schools are dropping physical education classes and assigning more homework, leaving less time for sports and physical activity. Newer communities often lack a central shopping area that people can walk to and many are built without sidewalks or bike paths, so people are forced to drive everywhere. For many people, hectic work and family schedules simply don't allow time for physical activities.

The eating habits of many families have also changed significantly over the past few decades. The variety of available foods has multiplied, and portion sizes in most restaurants have increased dramatically. Fast foods and packaged convenience foods that are high in fat, salt, and sugar often replace nutritious home-cooked meals and fresh fruits and vegetables, which are less loaded with calories. School lunches frequently offer high-calorie, high-fat foods such as pizza, french fries, and macaroni and cheese, along with sugary soft drinks and fruit drinks, and fail to offer nutritious choices such as low-fat milk, fruits, and vegetables. Many schools sell candy bars and other high-fat snacks in vending machines. Children, especially adolescents, need a lot of calories to fuel their growth and development, but when they are inactive, they end up taking in more calories than they burn and, as a result, they put on weight.

Is Your Child at Risk?

In a child who is genetically vulnerable to developing type 2 diabetes, being overweight is usually the stressor that brings it on. Excess weight, especially when it accumulates in the abdominal area, can make the cells become insensitive, or resistant, to the effects of the hormone insulin, which is responsible for helping glucose gain entrance into cells to be used for energy. To help the insensitive cells take in glucose and keep blood glucose steady, the pancreas produces more and more insulin. Eventually, however, the amount of insulin the pancreas is able to produce cannot compensate for the decreased insulin sensitivity of the cells, and glucose begins to build up in the blood, eventually leading to type 2 diabetes.

Children with type 2 diabetes are usually diagnosed during middle-to-late puberty because of the hormone changes that occur at that time. However, as children become more and more overweight and less active, more cases of type 2 diabetes may be diagnosed in children even before they reach puberty. The more risk factors your child has, the greater his or her chances of developing type 2 diabetes.

Children most at risk are those in families in which type 2 diabetes is present and who are significantly overweight and inactive. Genes have a major influence on the risk of type 2 diabetes—a child who has a parent or sibling with type 2 diabetes is two to six times more likely to develop type 2 diabetes than a child with no family history of the disease. If both parents have type 2 diabetes, the risk is increased even more. In the United States, Native American, Alaska Native, African American, and Hispanic American children have a significantly higher risk for type 2 diabetes than non-Hispanic whites; Hispanic Americans and non-Hispanic blacks are twice as likely as non-Hispanic whites to develop type 2 diabetes, and Native Americans and Alaskan Natives are three times as likely.

Less well understood are the following factors that can increase a child's risk of type 2 diabetes: being born to a mother who had diabetes during pregnancy (see page 205) and having a low birth weight. Exposure to diabetes before birth is one of the factors that doctors think play a role in the increase in type 2 diabetes among children. As more women develop gestational diabetes during pregnancy, increasing numbers of their children will be at risk for type 2 diabetes.

Being Overweight

In the United States, 9 million children over age 6 are obese (more than 20 percent over their ideal weight). About 30 percent of children and adolescents between the ages of 6 and 19 are overweight, and 15 percent are obese. In childhood, boys are more likely to be overweight than girls, but during adolescence the number of overweight or obese boys and girls is about equal.

Health Risks of Being Overweight

Being overweight is the major risk factor for type 2 diabetes as well as for high blood pressure. These common chronic disorders, which used to be rare among children, are occurring increasingly in American children and adolescents as a result of too little exercise and too many calories.

In the past three decades, childhood obesity has doubled in the United States among preschool children and teens and tripled among children between the ages of 6 and 11, trends that are expected to produce a combined epidemic of obesity and type 2 diabetes in children. If these trends continue, one in every three babies born today will develop type 2 diabetes at some time in his or her lifetime.

A child between the ages of 6 and 11 today has twice the risk of becoming overweight as a child the same age 20 years ago. Children who are very overweight usually have above-average blood pressure and heart rate, and children and teenagers who are overweight are more likely to stay overweight as adults. Overweight adults are at increased risk for type 2 diabetes, heart disease, high blood pressure, stroke, some types of cancer, and gallbladder disease.

Being overweight can also cause other health problems for children. Following are some of the health conditions that overweight children can experience:

- **High Blood Pressure**   As increasing numbers of American children become overweight, the number of children diagnosed with high blood pressure (see page 237) is also increasing. High blood pressure is nine times more common in children who are overweight than in children of normal weight. Without treatment, high blood pressure can cause long-term, often serious and irreversible health problems, including heart damage and stroke.

- **Bone and Joint Problems**   Excess weight puts extra stress on the hip and leg joints, and because children are still growing, this stress can cause abnormal turning of the lower leg inward or outward, bowed legs, or separation of the ball of the hip joint from the thigh bone (especially in boys).

- **Skin Disorders**   Overweight children are more likely than children of normal weight to experience heat rash, intertrigo (inflammation cause by skin rubbing against skin, especially in hot and humid weather), rashes, and acanthosis nigricans (see page 207).

- **Emotional Problems**   Because of the stigma associated with being overweight in our society, some children who are overweight have low self-esteem, a negative self-image, behavioral and learning problems, and depression, and can become withdrawn and isolated from their peers.

Overweight in children is a complex problem caused by the interaction of many factors including heredity, metabolism, behavior, environment, culture, and economic status. Behavior and environment may or may not be the major factors that cause a child to become overweight, but they represent the best ways to prevent and reverse it.

Because children grow at different rates, it is not always easy to tell if a child is overweight for his or her age. If you think that your child may be overweight, talk to his or her doctor. The doctor can measure your child's height and weight and determine if your child is in the

BMI for Children and Teens

Doctors use the body mass index (BMI) differently to evaluate weight in children and teens than in adults. Body fat changes as children grow, and girls and boys differ in body fat as they mature. For this reason, the BMI measurement in children is called BMI-for-age and is plotted on the traditional gender-specific growth charts from the Centers for Disease Control and Prevention (CDC) that pediatricians have used for years. Each of the CDC BMI-for-age gender-specific charts contains a series of curved lines indicating specific percentiles representing the average growth of children comparable in age and gender. Doctors use the following percentiles to determine if they are overweight or at risk of becoming overweight, are at a normal weight, or are underweight.

EVALUATING YOUR CHILD'S BMI

BMI-for-Age	Weight Assessment
At or higher than the 95th percentile	Overweight
Between the 85th and 95th percentiles	At risk of being overweight
Between the 5th and 85th percentiles	Normal weight
Under the 5th percentile	Underweight

healthy range for his or her age and sex. If your child is significantly overweight, the doctor will work with you to develop a plan to help your child reach a healthy weight. One of the things the doctor will recommend is to encourage your child to become much more physically active, so he or she is burning more calories.

Family History

A family history of type 2 diabetes is a strong influence on a child's risk of developing the disorder. Insulin resistance (see page 12), which is often the precursor to type 2 diabetes, is much more common in children with a family history of type 2 diabetes than in children without a family history of the disorder. Having a parent or a sibling with type 2 diabetes is an especially strong risk factor. Identical twins have identical genes. When one identical twin develops type 2 diabetes, the other twin has a 75 percent chance of also developing it. When one identical twin develops type 1 diabetes, the other twin has a 50 percent chance of developing it.

But it's good to keep in mind that although most children with type 2 diabetes have inherited genes that make them susceptible to developing the disease, having the genes does not mean that they are destined to develop it. Developing type 2 diabetes probably depends on both genetic and environmental factors. In the United States and other developed countries, these environmental factors include being overweight, getting too little exercise, and eating too much saturated fat and too little fiber. Countries that have not adopted a Western or urban lifestyle have a much lower incidence of type 2 diabetes.

Ethnic Background

Young people with type 2 diabetes belong to all ethnic groups, but the disorder is more common in some ethnic groups than in others. Native American children have the highest incidence of type 2 diabetes of all children in the United States, but children with an Hispanic American, African American, Asian, or Pacific Islander heritage also are at increased risk.

Adolescents now comprise about 15 percent of the US population. The racial and ethnic composition of the adolescent population in the United States is changing rapidly and is expected to become increasingly diverse in this century. In 1999, two-thirds of all adolescents were non-Hispanic whites but by 2050, experts predict that young Native Americans, Hispanic Americans, African Americans, and Asians will make up 56 percent of the adolescent population. Given the high risk of type 2 diabetes in these groups, the disorder is on track to become even more widespread if steps are not taken to reverse its primary causes: overweight, inactivity, and poor eating habits.

Native Americans

Type 2 diabetes among young people has been emerging as a major concern in Native American communities in the United States over the past 40 years. Because of their genetic susceptibility to type 2 diabetes, Native American adolescents, especially those from the Pima tribe in Arizona, have the highest incidence of type 2 diabetes in the world. The extraordinary rate of type 2 diabetes among young Native Americans raises concerns about the impact of diabetes on future generations. While the overall incidence of type 2 diabetes among Native Americans of all ages increased 46 percent during the 1990s, the largest increases occurred among adolescents ages 15 to 19—an 81 percent jump among males and 60 percent among females.

Hispanic Americans

Hispanic Americans represent the fastest-growing segment of the US population, and their average age is 10 years younger than that of the general population. This group has a high incidence of type 2 diabetes and tends to develop type 2 diabetes and its precursor, insulin resistance (see page 12), at younger ages than usual. To further complicate the problem, diabetes and insulin resistance remain undiagnosed in more than half of all Hispanic Americans who are affected.

African Americans

More than 3 million African Americans—1 out of 10—have type 2 diabetes; on average, this is twice the rate of that of non-Hispanic white Americans. African Americans with diabetes are more likely to develop diabetes complications (see chapter 13) and to experience greater disability from the complications than are non-Hispanic white Americans with diabetes.

The occurrence of gestational diabetes (diabetes that develops during pregnancy; see chapter 15) in African American women may be 50 to 80 percent higher than in non-Hispanic white women. A child whose mother had gestational diabetes during pregnancy is at increased risk of developing type 2 diabetes, which may partially explain the higher incidence of type 2 diabetes among African American children compared with non-Hispanic white children.

Asian Americans

Asian Americans' risk of type 2 diabetes in childhood and adolescence is not as high as that of some other minorities but is higher than that of non-Hispanic whites. Asian Americans seem to develop the disorder at a lower weight than other people. Japan has recently seen a dramatic rise in the occurrence of type 2 diabetes among school-age children—a sevenfold increase since 1976. The increase is even greater among children in junior high. Researchers think the increase can be explained by the detrimental changes in eating patterns and weight gain in young Japanese as they adopt a Western diet and lifestyle that includes fast foods and sugary soft drinks and less exercise.

In a similar way, the incidence of type 2 diabetes among Asians rises when they move to the United States or other Western countries or from rural areas to cities in their native country. This usually results from their giving up their traditional plant- and fish-based diet and eating foods with more animal protein, animal fats, and processed carbohydrates. The Western diet is also often higher in calories and lower in fiber, and the fat content is sometimes double that of the traditional Asian diet. To add to the problem, Asians are often exchanging their traditional lifestyle, characterized by lots of physical activity, for the much less active lifestyle that is common in Western countries. The move from rural areas to cities and suburbs results in a dramatic reduction in physical activity.

Eating Too Much

The diet of many American children can be summed up in two opposing phrases: too much and not enough. Many children are eating too much sugar, too much saturated and trans fats, and too much salt and not enough fiber-rich fruits, vegetables, and other complex carbohydrates (such as whole grains). Together, this lopsided diet and a sedentary lifestyle are the environmental factors that doctors often refer to as triggers for type 2 diabetes in children who have inherited genes that make them susceptible to the disorder.

Following is a list of some of the foods you should try to avoid giving your children, or give in very limited amounts. If you can manage to steer your children away from these foods, which tend to provide lots of calories but little nutrition, you will be taking a big step toward making your children healthier.

- **Sugary Soft Drinks** Sugary soft drinks contain about 8 teaspoons of sugar, or 150 calories, in a 12-ounce serving, making them a leading cause of weight gain in American children (and adults). Soft drinks are wasted or excess calories because they provide no essential nutrients.
- **French Fries** Deep-fried, often in harmful trans fats, french fries comprise a huge percentage of the unhealthy fats that many children consume regularly. They provide many calories and few nutrients.

- **Deep-fried Chicken Pieces**   Also frequently deep-fried in trans fats, chicken fingers and other fried fast foods are high in fat and salt.
- **Doughnuts**   They may taste good, but doughnuts are high in fat and sugar and have no nutritional value.
- **Snack Chips**   Many brands of potato and tortilla chips are made with trans fats and contain lots of salt.
- **Juice Drinks**   Drinks that contain less than 100 percent fruit juice provide mostly empty calories from sugar and few nutrients. It's much healthier to eat a piece of fruit, which contains fiber, than to drink fruit juice.
- **Chewy Fruit Snacks**   Don't let the word *fruit* fool you—these treats are candy in disguise. They are full of added sugar and they stick to the teeth, where they can promote cavities.
- **Hot Dogs**   High in fat and salt, hot dogs provide little protein. Cut-up hot dogs are a choking hazard for children under the age of 3.
- **Processed Deli Meats**   Most deli meats contain excessive amounts of salt, and many are high in fat. If your children insist on eating sandwich meats, buy the low-fat or fat-free and reduced-sodium varieties.

Instead of serving your children these unhealthy foods, provide a variety of low-fat protein sources, such as lean meats, poultry, and fish; fresh fruits and vegetables; and whole-grain cereals and breads. Include low-fat milk, yogurt, and cheese daily unless your child is lactose intolerant (has a reaction to the sugar lactose in dairy products; see page 227). For dessert, offer fresh fruit, dried fruit (but only in moderation because, ounce for ounce, dried fruit is much higher in calories than fresh fruit), fruit smoothies, frozen fruit bars, or reduced-fat or low-fat frozen yogurt.

Being Inactive

A child's body is made for physical activity, but American children are becoming less and less physically active and, as a result, are getting fatter. In addition to helping control weight, regular physical activity during childhood and adolescence improves strength and endurance, helps build strong muscles and bones, reduces anxiety and stress, improves blood pressure and cholesterol levels, and may increase self-esteem. Positive experiences with physical activity at a young age also help lay the foundation for a pattern of regular physical activity throughout life. More than one-third of all high school students fail to engage in regular vigorous physical activity, and less than a third of high school students attend physical education classes in school on a daily basis. The older a child is, the less likely he or she is to engage in regular physical activity.

Here are some things you can do to help promote physical activity in your child's school and in your community:

- Talk to your child's school about scheduling more active time for students.
- Ask if the school will allow the building to be used for non-school-related physical activities after hours.
- Sign up your child for physical activities and sports with the local park district, Boy or Girl Scouts, 4H, or Boys and Girls Clubs.
- Talk to community planners about providing safe and active places for kids to play.
- Volunteer to help create or fix up local playgrounds.

Physical activity, done on a routine basis, helps burn the extra calories that many children are consuming every time they eat a high-calorie snack. The bottom line: regular physical activity helps keep kids from gaining those excess pounds that can place them at risk of becoming overweight and developing type 2 diabetes.

Having a Mother Who Had Diabetes during Pregnancy

If a woman has diabetes or develops high blood sugar during pregnancy (gestational diabetes; see chapter 15), her child has an increased risk of obesity and of developing type 2 diabetes at some time in his or her life.

In addition to inheriting a tendency to develop diabetes, children whose mother had diabetes also seem to be susceptible by being exposed to a "diabetic environment" before birth. This does not mean that a baby from a diabetes pregnancy will be born with diabetes or necessarily develop it as a child. Lifestyle factors such as eating a healthy diet, getting regular exercise, maintaining a healthy weight, and keeping blood pressure normal can help a child avoid type 2 diabetes.

Low Birth Weight

Doctors have linked low birth weight to future risk of type 2 diabetes, although they do not fully understand exactly how the two are related. Several years ago, researchers found that people who had a heart attack or diabetes or who were obese in their 60s and 70s were more likely to have been of lower-than-average weight at birth. Then it was learned from growth charts kept during school years that people who had been small at birth but had grown rapidly as children and become overweight during adolescence were the most likely to be obese or have heart disease or diabetes later in life. More recent research suggests that people whose birth weight is less than expected for their length at birth (thin babies) may be the most vulnerable.

As the number of premature babies who are very small at birth and surviving increases, there is concern about their future health risks. However, while the birth weight of premature babies may be very low, these babies are not necessarily small for the time in pregnancy at which they were born. The long-term risks of obesity, heart disease, and diabetes in premature babies are not known.

Puberty

Puberty is a critical time in the development of type 2 diabetes in at-risk children. In all children, the first stages of puberty cause changes in hormone levels that make the cells less sensitive to insulin. In most adolescents, this decreased sensitivity, or resistance, to insulin does not cause problems. However, in susceptible children who are already insulin resistant from being overweight and inactive, the added insulin resistance of puberty can bring on type 2 diabetes.

Symptoms, Diagnosis, and Treatment

Type 2 diabetes can be difficult to diagnose early in children because it frequently produces no symptoms. If your child's doctor suspects that your child has type 2 diabetes, he or she will order tests to make an accurate diagnosis and to distinguish it from type 1 diabetes. Once diagnosed with type 2 diabetes, children and teenagers need help from their parents, teachers, and health-care providers to develop the coping skills necessary to manage and adapt to life with a chronic disorder, including establishing healthy eating and exercise habits.

Symptoms

It can be hard to tell if a child has type 2 diabetes because, as in adults, it seldom causes symptoms. For this reason, the disorder can go undiagnosed for some time. Blood tests are needed to make a diagnosis. Because there is no widespread screening for type 2 diabetes in children, it's important to talk to your child's doctor about testing if you think your child may be at risk. This is especially important if you have a family history of type 2 diabetes and your child is substantially overweight.

Acanthosis Nigricans

Acanthosis nigricans is a skin disorder that is common in children with type 2 diabetes. The disorder is characterized by dark, velvety skin in the body folds and creases. The affected skin ranges from light brown to black and appears most frequently on the neck and knuckles and in the armpits and groin. Sometimes the lips, palms, soles of the feet, and other sites are affected. Acanthosis nigricans most often occurs in children who are overweight; it is less common in overweight adults.

Doctors think that high levels of insulin and insulin resistance contribute to the development of acanthosis nigricans. The excess insulin somehow stimulates the skin to pigment abnormally. The most effective treatment for acanthosis nigricans is to reduce the level of insulin in the bloodstream by following a special diet and losing weight.

Polycystic Ovarian Syndrome

Polycystic ovarian syndrome (see page 29) is a condition characterized by the presence of numerous small cysts in the ovaries. The condition often appears during late adolescence in susceptible girls. In these girls, the level of the male hormone testosterone is slightly elevated and produces many of the syndrome's characteristic symptoms, including the accumulation of fat around the abdomen. Other symptoms include irregular menstrual cycles, a failure to ovulate, and excess facial hair.

Polycystic ovarian syndrome is strongly linked to insulin resistance and carries an increased risk of type 2 diabetes.

Diagnosis

Because puberty normally makes the cells less sensitive to insulin, doctors usually begin to test children who are at high risk for type 2 diabetes at around age 10 or at the beginning of puberty (if puberty occurs earlier than age 10). The doctor may test your child for the disorder at an even younger age if your child weighs more than 20 percent over the ideal weight range for his or her age and height or has a body mass index (BMI; see page 35) over the 85th percentile among children of his or her age and height. Other factors that could make a doctor test early include a strong family history of type 2 diabetes and being of African American, Hispanic American, Native American, Asian, or Pacific Islander descent. The doctor will also suspect the presence of insulin resistance or type 2 diabetes if your child has acanthosis nigricans (see previous page), polycystic ovarian syndrome (see page 29), high blood pressure (see page 238), or abnormal cholesterol (see page 94) because of the close association these conditions have with type 2 diabetes.

Doctors usually diagnose type 2 diabetes in a child by evaluating a child's weight, symptoms, family history, and the results of a thorough physical examination. Your child's doctor will assess your child's weight by comparing it with the normal percentile ranges in weight and height for children the same age. The doctor will consider your child to be overweight if he or she is heavier than 85 percent of children of the same age and height. If your child is overweight, the doctor will perform a thorough physical examination to determine how overweight the child is and will rule out any physical conditions, such as an underactive thyroid gland, that could be contributing to the weight problem. In rare cases, some genetic disorders can cause obesity, so the doctor will also want to rule these out.

The doctor may look for signs of an eating disorder, such as binge eating or bulimia (the use of vomiting or laxatives to eliminate calories and avoid weight gain). Depression can also cause children to overeat compulsively. Eating disorders require a thorough psychological evaluation by a mental health professional and treatment because, without treatment, they can undermine a child's weight-control program and lead to serious health problems.

The doctor will also check for other treatable physical problems that are associated with being overweight—including joint problems, sleep apnea (periodic cessation of breathing during sleep), and polycystic ovarian syndrome. These problems will be improved with weight loss, but they sometimes require treatment.

The results of the usual diabetes tests (see page 90), such as the fasting blood glucose or the oral glucose tolerance tests, may be enough to indicate a diagnosis of type 2 diabetes. Children are usually diagnosed with type 2 diabetes if their fasting plasma glucose exceeds 126 mg/dL or if their glucose level is higher than 200 mg/dL when checked randomly, 2 hours after eating a meal, or during a glucose tolerance test.

If doubt remains, the doctor may order additional blood tests such as a fasting insulin test, an insulin C-peptide test, and an autoantibody test. The fasting insulin test measures the amount of insulin in the blood. The insulin C-peptide test can determine if any insulin is being produced by the body. The autoantibody test helps distinguish type 2 diabetes from type 1 by identifying antibodies that attack the islet cells in the pancreas; the presence of a high level of these antibodies is an indication of type 1 diabetes.

Treatment

The main goals in treating a child with type 2 diabetes are keeping blood sugar levels as close to normal as possible and preventing complications. If your child has type 2 diabetes, he or she needs to be taught how to manage the disorder at home. Your child's doctor will help you choose a program that has a team of educators experienced in working with children with type 2 diabetes, including a dietitian, a nurse, a social worker, and an exercise specialist. You and your child will be taught how to monitor his or her blood sugar levels, develop an exercise program, and plan meals that meet treatment goals but also take into account your child's food preferences. If your child needs to take medication, you will learn how to take it and about its effects. Check to see if your local hospital has a pediatric center with Certified Diabetes Educators on staff and whose programs have met the National Standards for Diabetes Self-Management Education set by the American Diabetes Association.

Young people with type 2 diabetes face tough challenges when presented with treatment options. Because children often don't have any symptoms, families may have a hard time acknowledging that the child has a potentially serious health problem. Even after a diagnosis of type 2 diabetes, some families find it difficult to cope with the magnitude of the changes required in their daily routine and to fully support the child's treatment regimen. Before treatment starts, get your child prepared and motivated to make the changes needed to manage his or her blood sugar, eat right, and exercise more.

Because of the high level of motivation demanded of a child or an adolescent with diabetes to follow his or her treatment regimen, treatment is most likely to be successful when the entire family makes it a team effort. Family members should share their concerns with the doctor, diabetes educator, dietitian, and any other health-care providers working with the child so they can help in the day-to-day management of the disorder. Teachers, school nurses, counselors, coaches, day-care providers, and other people in your community who are in contact with your child can provide information, support, and guidance to help you cope with your caregiving responsibilities.

Weight Control

For children with type 2 diabetes who are overweight, doctors focus weight-control efforts on three areas: diet, exercise, and behavior changes. You as a parent are an integral part of your child's success in this effort, which will include targeted goals of increasing physical activity and reducing consumption of high-fat and high-calorie foods. Doctors usually first recommend a weight-maintenance strategy that involves replacing unhealthy behaviors with healthy ones, primarily increasing physical activity and eating a nutritious diet. Over time, it is hoped that the child's BMI (see page 200) will gradually decline as he or she grows in height. The younger your child is when he or she develops healthy eating habits, the more likely he or she is to eat healthfully throughout life.

In children over age 7 who are significantly overweight (a BMI of 35 or more or a BMI-for-age at or above the 95th percentile), weight loss of 1 to 2 pounds per week may be recommended. Before recommending weight loss, a doctor will usually evaluate the benefits and risks of weight loss against the severity of any weight-related health problems a child has.

Overweight children need support, acceptance, and encouragement from their parents and other family members. Most overweight children perceive social exclusion to be the most hurtful consequence of

The Traffic-Light Diet

One popular weight-control approach that is easily understood by young children is the traffic-light diet. The traffic-light diet is a practical eating plan that provides 900 to 1,300 calories per day, concentrating on foods that boost the nutrient content of the diet. The traffic-light diet teaches children good nutrition by relating specific foods to the three signals on a traffic light: green foods ("Go!") provide lots of nutrients and can be eaten in unlimited quantities; yellow foods ("Caution") contain only a moderate amount of nutrients for the number of calories and should be eaten in moderation; and red foods ("Stop!") supply few nutrients but lots of calories (because of a high fat or sugar content) and should be avoided or strictly limited.

The traffic-light diet has been found to produce considerable weight reduction in overweight children. The diet increases a child's intake of important nutrients, such as protein, calcium, iron, vitamin A, and the B vitamins, and reduces the intake of harmful fats and sugars. Overweight school-age children who follow the traffic-light diet seem to lose their taste for high-fat, sugary foods and acquire a taste for low-fat, less-sweet foods. Just as important, children who follow the diet tend to stay in the normal weight range for their age and height for 5 to 10 years after starting the diet, provided they stay physically active.

their being overweight. Being shunned by peers can often lead to low self-esteem and depression. To counteract this effect, let your child know you love and appreciate him or her no matter what his or her weight. An overweight child probably knows better than anyone else that he or she has a weight problem. Listen to your child's concerns about his or her weight. Encourage your child to exercise with other children who also need to lose weight—they'll feel comfortable together and they can reinforce one another's good behavior.

Here are a few things you can do to help your child reach a healthy weight:

- Don't force your child to eat when he or she is not hungry—it's fine if your child doesn't finish everything on his or her plate. Eating when you're not hungry is a major cause of weight gain.

- Don't promise a sweet dessert or other high-calorie treat as a reward for finishing a meal, because it will teach your child that sweets are more desirable than more nutritious foods. Serve fruit for dessert and offer special activities and time with you as rewards for good behavior.

- Don't eat at fast-food restaurants more than once a month.
- Monitor your child's TV viewing and computer time and limit these sedentary activities to 1 hour a day. Encourage your child to engage in physical activity for at least 2 hours a day.
- Focus on your child's health and positive qualities, not on his or her weight. Find reasons to praise good behaviors.
- Set daily meal and snack times and stick to them as much as you can.
- Try not to make your child feel different from other people. Focus on gradually changing your family's exercise and eating habits.
- Provide only healthy food choices and suggest only healthy activities. "Do you want an apple or a pear?" "Do you want to ride your bike or take a walk?"
- Be a good role model. If your child sees you enjoying healthy foods and being physically active, he or she is more likely to do the same.
- Stay consistent and be firm. Don't occasionally give in to requests for unhealthy foods, because such periodic acquiescence can reinforce unwanted behavior.

Restrict your child's calorie intake by limiting calorie-dense junk food, sweets, and sugary soft drinks so your child's basic diet remains nutritious. It should include all of the recommended dietary allowances for vitamins, minerals, and protein and contain a variety of foods from the following groups: whole grains (breads, cereals, and pasta), fruits, vegetables, lean sources of protein, and dairy products (if your child isn't lactose intolerant; see page 227). Teach your child that weight control will be a lifelong goal, as it is for many people. Here are some guidelines for helping to make your child's efforts to control his or her weight successful:

- Encourage your child to eat slowly.
- Eat meals together as a family as often as possible.
- Cut down on the amount of fat and calories in your family's diet.
- Don't withhold food as punishment.
- Encourage your child to drink water and to avoid drinks with added sugars, such as sugary soft drinks, fruit juice and fruit drinks, and sports drinks.

- Try to have your child eat at least 5 to 10 servings of fruits and vegetables each day.
- Serve healthy snacks such as fruit and cut-up fresh vegetables.
- Stock the refrigerator with fat-free or low-fat milk and fresh fruits and vegetables instead of sugary soft drinks or snacks that are high in fat, calories, or added sugars.
- Discourage eating while watching TV, playing video games, or reading.
- Serve your child a healthy breakfast every day.
- Follow the government's Dietary Guidelines for healthy eating (see page 116).

If your child has developed serious complications such as sleep apnea (the periodic cessation of breathing during sleep) from being over-weight, rapid weight loss may be required. In this case, the doctor may refer your child to a pediatric obesity center run by doctors and other health-care workers who have experience managing quick, safe weight loss. Your child will be given a special diet and exercise program along with any needed medication. In rare cases, weight-loss surgery (see page 103) may be recommended.

Meal Planning

A meal plan tailored to a child's needs and preferences is an essential component of treatment for type 2 diabetes. The diabetes meal plan emphasizes eating nutritious foods for healthy growth and for keeping blood glucose levels in the target range. You and your child will learn how different types of food—especially carbohydrates such as white breads, pasta, and rice—can affect blood sugar. You will also learn about portion size, the appropriate amount of daily calories based on your child's age, and how to make healthy food choices at meal and snack times. Family support is essential for your child to successfully follow the meal plan. Scheduling regular meal times is also important, especially if your child is taking insulin.

Your child's meal plan should be developed by a dietitian or a diabetes educator who has experience planning meals for children with type 2 diabetes. The dietitian will emphasize how important it is for the entire family to eat healthfully so the child with diabetes doesn't feel deprived of family favorites. When planning your child's diet, the dietitian or diabetes educator will take into account your family's lifestyle and cultural preferences.

Exercise

For overweight children, increased physical activity is an integral part in helping them reach a healthy weight. Exercise not only burns calories, it also boosts the sensitivity of the cells to insulin, helping to keep blood glucose in the healthy range. An exercise counselor who has experience working with children with type 2 diabetes can help your child and other family members develop a sensible exercise program that takes into account their interests and abilities.

Your child should get at least 1 hour of moderately vigorous exercise every day. If your child does not have recess or physical education classes at school or if he or she uses the time in sedentary activities, try to block out 10- or 15-minute periods for exercise in the morning and after school. The more physically active your child is—that is, following a routine of physical activity that lasts longer or is more intense—the greater the health benefits. Jogging, stair climbing, swimming laps, and singles tennis are good aerobic exercises.

In addition to helping with weight loss, regular physical activity helps control blood sugar, especially in children and adolescents with type 2 diabetes. For more about exercise, see page 234.

Blood Sugar Monitoring

Your child may have to check his or her blood glucose levels regularly with a blood glucose meter (see page 139), preferably one with built-in memory. The doctor or nurse can teach your child how to use the meter properly and how often to check his or her blood glucose level. Blood glucose meter results show whether blood sugar levels are in the target range, too high, or too low. Your child should keep a journal, recording blood glucose results that the doctor can use to evaluate the effectiveness of the treatment plan and recommend any necessary changes. Measuring blood sugar on a regular basis can help you and your child understand the effects that particular foods, physical activity, and stress have on your child's blood sugar.

You will have to use a finger-pricking device (lancet) to draw a drop of blood from your child's finger. Adjustable lancets are especially good for young children who have sensitive skin, because you don't need to prick too deeply. Remember to use a new lancet for each test. Place the drop of blood on a test strip and insert the strip into the blood glucose meter. Different meters measure blood sugar in different ways, so you can't always compare the results from different meters. It doesn't matter which type of meter you use as long as you always use the same meter. Bring the meter with you to each of your child's visits to the doctor. The doctor can record the information from the meter and keep it in your child's medical records.

Occasionally, the blood glucose meter may show that your child's sugar levels are too low, a potentially serious condition called hypoglycemia (see page 159). Hypoglycemia occurs primarily in children with type 2 diabetes who are taking diabetes medication or insulin. Hypoglycemia can sometimes occur during exercise, so it's especially important to watch for symptoms. The longer and more vigorously your child exercises, the more watchful you need to be. If your child is taking medication or insulin, be sure to tell your child's coach and teammates about your child's diabetes and make sure they know how to treat low blood sugar.

Medications

When a child's blood sugar reaches a certain level, or when weight loss, diet, and exercise have not lowered blood sugar sufficiently, a doctor will usually prescribe either metformin pills or insulin injections, which are the only medications approved for treating type 2 diabetes in

Diabetes Self-Care: How Old Should Your Child Be?

Some children are more mature than others the same age, but in general, you can expect your child to be able to follow directions well enough to take care of at least some aspects of his or her diabetes care at the following ages:

Age	Task
4 years	Can be cooperative when you need to do a fingerstick test or give an insulin shot
8 years	Can perform a fingerstick test of blood sugar, with supervision
13 years	Can monitor his or her own blood sugar (unless hypoglycemic); can administer insulin with supervision

At any age, children with diabetes will probably need help to perform a blood glucose test when their blood sugar level is low. Most children need to be reminded to eat or drink something during a period of low blood sugar, and you should not leave them unsupervised until they do.

children. Your child should take any diabetes medication exactly as the doctor prescribes. You, your child's doctor, and the school nurse can all help ensure that your child learns how to take the medications correctly. Some children or teens with type 2 diabetes need to take diabetes medications or insulin shots—or both—at regular times each day. Your child always needs to balance his or her medication with food intake and physical activity.

Oral Medications

There are several types of oral drugs that doctors prescribe for treating type 2 diabetes in adults. These drugs have been developed for and tested in adults. Because the incidence of type 2 diabetes in children is still relatively low, few studies have been done to test the safety and effectiveness of diabetes drugs in children, and only one of these drugs (metformin) has been approved by the Food and Drug Administration (FDA) for use in children. Metformin is an oral medication that has been used for about 40 years for treating type 2 diabetes in adults and was approved in 2001 for treating type 2 diabetes in children. In the future, additional effective medications will be available for treating children with type 2 diabetes.

Metformin improves blood sugar control by boosting insulin sensitivity in the liver and reducing the liver's production of glucose. When effective, metformin keeps blood sugar levels in a safe range without causing weight gain in children.

The most common side effects of metformin are nausea, loss of appetite, diarrhea, intestinal gas, and a metallic taste in the mouth. These side effects affect 10 to 15 percent of people who take the medication. Lactic acidosis, the buildup of lactic acid (a by-product of the breakdown of carbohydrates) in the body, is a very rare but life-threatening side effect of metformin. But lactic acidosis is more likely to occur in people who have heart, kidney, or liver failure, which are rare in children with diabetes.

A child should stop taking metformin if he or she develops any illness that causes vomiting or diarrhea or any condition that leads to dehydration. The medication should also be stopped before a child undergoes medical imaging tests requiring a dye (contrast agent). Because metformin can be passed to a fetus during pregnancy, doctors may prescribe insulin to adolescent girls with type 2 diabetes who engage in unprotected sexual intercourse and, therefore, could become pregnant.

Because type 2 diabetes develops and progresses in children in much the same way it does in adults, most doctors do not want to exclude children from the benefits of diabetes medications—controlling blood sugar levels and preventing diabetes complications. Experience with adults who have type 2 diabetes shows that over time blood sugar control becomes more difficult with single medications and frequently requires the addition of another medication, either one taken by mouth or insulin injections. Because children who have type 2 diabetes may need to start taking medication earlier in life than a person diagnosed with the disorder as an adult, strict observance of diet and exercise recommendations becomes all the more important, to postpone the time when medication must be taken.

Insulin

If lifestyle changes and oral glucose-lowering medication do not adequately control your child's blood sugar, he or she may need to begin taking insulin injections. Insulin injections are given into the layer of tissue between the muscle and the skin called the subcutaneous (under the skin) layer. Injecting insulin into this layer ensures that it will be absorbed at a steady rate, which helps keep blood sugar levels steady.

Subcutaneous tissue is present throughout the body, but some sites are better than others for giving insulin because they are away from large blood vessels and nerves. The best places for injecting insulin are in the upper, outside part of the arm; the front and sides of the thighs; the buttocks; the back, just above the waist; and the abdomen (except the areas around the navel and the waist).

The injection site needs to be changed frequently because repeated injections into the same site could injure sensitive tissue and reduce insulin absorption. The doctor or the nurse will show you and your child exactly how to give insulin injections and tell you how frequently to give them and how to rotate injection sites.

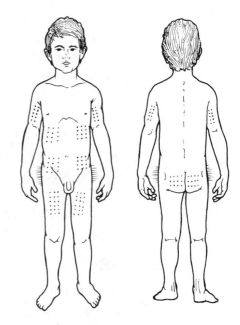

Where to Inject Insulin
If your child needs to take insulin, use this drawing to find the best places on the body to inject it. Rotate the injection sites often to minimize tissue injury because injury from repeated injections can inhibit the absorption of insulin. Common injection sites are the upper arms, abdomen, thighs, and buttocks.

Living with Type 2 Diabetes

Diabetes presents challenges for children. They have to pay careful attention to their diet, monitor their blood sugar levels, take diabetes medication or insulin, and deal with high or low blood sugar. Your child may sometimes feel that diabetes makes it impossible to lead a normal life. While your child's daily routine is different now from what it was before he or she developed diabetes, your family can still have a normal life by making diabetes care part of the family's daily routine. Let your child take care of his or her diabetes as much as possible, depending on his or her age. Taking personal responsibility for their diabetes care helps children become independent and prepares them to take on greater responsibility for the disorder as they grow up.

Try not to let diabetes become the focal point of your child's life; let him or her take part in as many interesting and fun activities as possible. Depending on the severity of your child's condition, simple things such as going to a birthday party, playing sports, or staying overnight with friends can require careful planning. Your child may need to take insulin or oral medication every day. He or she may also have to check blood glucose levels several times during the day and remember to make the right food choices. These tasks can make school-age children feel overly burdened and different from their classmates. Such problems often intensify during adolescence.

Special Occasions

Having diabetes shouldn't prevent your child from having as much fun as any other child on special occasions. Some advance planning can enable a child with diabetes to take part in most activities on holidays and other special occasions, such as pizza days at school, class parties, sleepovers, and birthday parties. Here are some basic guidelines for helping your child participate in and enjoy special occasions:

- Contact the event's planner and ask what food will be served and when.

- Find out what physical activities are planned. Your child may have to test his or her blood sugar level before, during, and after activities if the activities are vigorous.
- Figure out the exchanges or "food choice values" for the food being served, or ask the dietitian to help you do this.
- You may have to substitute different food groups to fit party foods into your child's meal plan. For example:

    2 milk choices = 1 starch choice + 1 protein choice

    1 starch choice = 1½ fruits and vegetables choice

    1 fruits and vegetables choice = 1 sugar choice

    2 starch choices = 3 sugar choices

- If there will be lots of physical activity, your child may need some extra food or a change in his or her insulin dose.

Family Relationships

After being diagnosed with diabetes, children often notice changes in the way their parents and siblings relate to them. You may worry more about your child, especially when he or she is away from home, and your other children may resent the special attention their sibling with diabetes is getting. Because siblings sometimes initially fear that diabetes is contagious and they will develop it too, try to assure them that diabetes is not like the common cold and is impossible to get from another person. Any changes in attitude by family members can trigger many conflicting emotions in a child with diabetes, from anger to frustration and anxiety about the future. These feelings are normal. You can help your child get through the hard times by always being there for him or her. Listen whenever he or she needs to talk.

You should also be sure you give your other children attention. Plan activities with each of your children that you both enjoy. These special times can help minimize their insecurities and make them more sensitive to their sibling with diabetes.

Diabetes affects the entire family, so get your whole family involved. To take the pressure off one parent, both parents should learn how to check blood sugar levels, understand blood sugar test results, and manage low and high blood sugar episodes. The more encouragement and help your child has from the rest of the family, the easier it will be for him or her to live normally with type 2 diabetes.

Hiring a Babysitter

All parents need to hire a babysitter from time to time. Make sure any babysitters you use know your child has diabetes, and familiarize them with your child's needs. Try to find a sitter who has taken a general course in babysitting from a local hospital or the American Red Cross. To acquaint the sitter with your child's eating and exercise routine, have him or her spend time with your child at least once when you are home before he or she stays alone with your child. Here are some tips to help make sure your child's needs are met:

- Write out a schedule of when your child needs to eat and the foods he or she should and should not eat. Tell the sitter to follow the schedule exactly.

- Do the same thing for exercise, specifying when and how much physical activity to allow. Ask the sitter to minimize TV time.

- Tell your sitter what to do if your children who do not have diabetes ask to have candy or sweets that your diabetic child can't have.

- Instruct the sitter to give all the children some special attention, not just the child with diabetes.

- Tell the sitter to call you immediately if your child with diabetes refuses to eat.

- If your child is treated with insulin, briefly describe the symptoms of low blood sugar so the sitter can recognize them, and tell him or her what to do to treat them.

- Give the sitter your cell phone number or the number at the location where you will be. In a true emergency, tell the sitter to call 911 first and then to call you.

Emotional Difficulties

For any child with type 2 diabetes, learning to cope with the disease is a huge challenge. Having a chronic illness such as diabetes can bring on emotional and behavioral problems because the disorder can make children feel different from their peers. If your child is overweight, he or she may be troubled by both the diabetes and being overweight. Overweight children are sometimes shunned by peers of normal weight and may be ridiculed or bullied at school. If your child is being bullied, get help. Talk to your child's teachers and the school principal and ask them to look into the situation. Tell your child to get immediate help from an adult when he or she is confronted by a bully.

Having diabetes is stressful for both the child and his or her entire family. Stay alert for signs of depression, difficulty coping, or the eating disorder bulimia (characterized by bingeing and purging, or eating large amounts and then self-inducing vomiting or using laxatives to eliminate the calories). If you notice any problems, get appropriate treatment for your child right away. Talking to a social worker or a psychologist can help a child or a teenager who has been diagnosed with type 2 diabetes—and his or her family—learn how to adjust to the many lifestyle changes needed to stay healthy.

While all parents should talk to their children about avoiding tobacco, alcohol, and illegal drugs, this conversation is especially important for children who have diabetes. Smoking and diabetes each increase the risk of heart disease and circulation problems later in life and the combination of the two can be especially dangerous. Binge drinking can cause hypoglycemia (low blood sugar) in people who are taking insulin; hypoglycemia has symptoms that can be mistaken for intoxication, preventing your child from getting appropriate and potentially lifesaving treatment. In people who are taking metformin, binge drinking increases the risk of lactic acidosis. Local support groups made up of children and teens with diabetes can give your child positive role models as well as provide group activities with other children who share the same experiences and concerns.

You may find that your anxiety level increases as you think about the possible consequences of your child's diabetes. Some parents worry that diabetes could affect their child's ability to learn, but studies have shown that children with diabetes perform as well academically as other children their age. You may be concerned about diabetes complications such as eye, kidney, heart, blood vessel, and nerve diseases (see chapter 13). Children seem to be protected from these complications during childhood, but persistent high blood sugar levels during childhood and adolescence raise their risk of having these complications in early adulthood—at much younger ages than people who develop type 2 diabetes later in life. Keeping your child's blood sugar levels as close to normal as possible can help prevent or delay future complications.

Diabetes Camps

Special overnight and summer day camps for children with diabetes are available throughout the United States and in many other parts of the world. These camps allow children with diabetes to have a camping experience in a safe environment that meets their needs for a special diet, blood sugar monitoring, and physical activity. Equally important is the chance for young people with diabetes to meet and share their experiences, while acquiring the skills needed to take greater responsibility for their condition.

As a parent of a child with diabetes, you are sure to have many health and safety concerns—from nutrition to medical care—about sending your child with diabetes away from home to camp. At diabetes camps, the counselors have been trained to deal with such concerns, and they can manage any emergency that may occur. Camp counselors know exactly how to provide the right nutrition, blood sugar checking, and exercise to manage their campers' conditions so they can relax and have fun.

Managing Low and High Blood Sugar

Keeping blood sugar levels within your child's target range is the goal of diabetes control, but extreme rises or falls in blood sugar can sometimes occur. Talk with your child's doctor about how you and your child should deal with these possible problems and then teach your child how to handle them.

Low Blood Sugar

Blood sugar levels can sometimes drop too low, a condition called hypoglycemia (see page 159). The condition occurs only in children taking insulin. Taking too much insulin, missing a meal or a snack, or exercising too long or too vigorously can cause hypoglycemia. Your child's brain relies on blood glucose as its primary source of fuel, and too little glucose can reduce the brain's ability to work properly. The initial symptoms of low blood sugar are nervousness, shakiness, irritability, and confusion, which resemble the symptoms of alcohol intoxication. If blood sugar falls lower, your child can lose consciousness, develop seizures, or go into a coma. Treat the low blood sugar right away by having your child consume something that contains sugar, such as orange juice, pancake syrup, milk, or a piece of hard candy.

High Blood Sugar

Blood glucose levels can sometimes rise too high, producing a condition called hyperglycemia. Forgetting to take diabetes medication on time, eating too much, and getting too little exercise can bring on hyperglycemia. Being sick, such as having a cold with a fever, can also raise blood sugar levels.

Unlike low blood sugar, high blood sugar usually comes on gradually, taking hours or days to develop. Blood glucose levels that are very elevated can make a child feel fatigued and thirsty and increase his or her need to urinate, but not all children with hyperglycemia have symptoms. Over time, excessively high blood sugar levels can lead to serious health problems and can damage the eyes, kidneys, nerves, blood vessels, and gums. If your child's blood sugar level keeps rising, his or her kidneys will produce more and more urine, which could lead to dehydration. Severe dehydration can cause coma and even death.

If your child has any of the symptoms of high blood sugar, treat it with medication or insulin immediately to prevent it from becoming an emergency. Take the following steps to help prevent your child from developing high blood sugar:

- Check your child's blood sugar often, especially if he or she is sick, eating too much, exercising too little, or has forgotten to take his or her diabetes medication.
- Call your child's doctor if episodes of high blood sugar are frequent or last longer than 2 or 3 hours. The doctor may need to change your child's medication or insulin dosage.
- Urge your child to drink plenty of water to prevent dehydration.

Preventing Type 2 Diabetes in Children

Preventing type 2 diabetes in children involves controlling a number of lifestyle factors aimed primarily at keeping children from becoming overweight. The most important concerns are to provide a healthy diet for your child, from the beginning of life, and make sure your child is physically active. Have your child's blood pressure checked at every well-child visit because high blood pressure often accompanies type 2 diabetes. It's also important to minimize the stress in your child's life; stress may contribute to the development of diabetes by raising levels of the stress hormone cortisol and by leading a child to overeat.

Maintaining a Healthy Weight

Being overweight during childhood and adolescence is strongly linked with being overweight as an adult. But overweight children who are still growing may not need to be put on a weight-loss diet—they may be able to stop or reduce their rate of weight gain and "grow into" their weight as they grow in height. But if your child is severely overweight, his or her doctor may recommend and closely supervise a weight-loss diet (see page 210). Even for extremely overweight children, weight loss should be gradual. Crash diets and diet pills can adversely affect a child's growth, and are rarely recommended by doctors. Like adults, children who lose weight are likely to regain it unless they are motivated to change their eating habits and activity level for life.

If your child is overweight, a simple, healthy approach to weight maintenance can be effective. Remove all junk food from your home and encourage your child to become more active. Don't let your children eat while watching TV, reading, or riding in the car because they will not be paying attention to the amount of food they're eating and are more likely to overeat. Teach your children to eat only when sitting down at the kitchen or dining room table and to eat only when they're hungry. Once these good eating habits become established, they can keep your child healthy as he or she grows and can reduce the risk of type 2 diabetes, heart disease, and other common chronic disorders later in life.

Healthy Foods from the Start

Breast milk is the healthiest source of nutrition for babies in their first year of life—it contains the precise amount of fatty acids, the milk sugar lactose, water, and amino acids that babies need for digestion, brain development, and growth. Breast-fed babies tend to have fewer infections because they receive their mother's infection-fighting antibodies in the breast milk. In addition, no babies are allergic to breast milk.

Breast-fed babies are less likely to be overweight than bottle-fed babies, and breast-feeding may reduce a child's risk of becoming overweight during puberty, between ages 9 and 14 years. Breast-fed babies learn to regulate their appetite because they stop nursing when they are full. In addition, breast-fed babies have lower levels of insulin, so their body may store less fat. These factors may help reduce a child's risk of developing type 2 diabetes later in life. Doctors recommend breast-feeding during a child's first year of life, with breast milk being a baby's sole source of nutrition during the first six months, before solid foods are introduced. By the time your child is a year old, he or she will be able to drink cow's milk.

You also get benefits from breast-feeding. Breast-feeding helps you lose the extra weight you gained during pregnancy because you're burning more calories. And in addition to reducing your risk of breast cancer, breast-feeding for longer than six months may reduce your risk of developing type 2 diabetes.

Instilling healthy eating habits early in life can help your child acquire a preference for healthy foods. Offer your child a variety of nutritious foods, including fruits and vegetables—including those you don't like. Avoid prepared baby foods that are high in salt, and don't add salt to the homemade foods you give your baby. Serve whole-grain breads, bagels, and pancakes instead of white-flour products. An occasional cookie is fine, but don't give your baby pastries or candy during the first few of years of life. Never give a baby or a toddler sugary soft drinks because they are one of the main sources of non-nutritious calories that make many American children overweight.

Children under the age of 2 need fat in their diet for proper growth and brain development. But when your child is between the ages of 2 and 3, that amount should be gradually reduced until he or she is consuming 25 to 30 percent of total calories from fat, which is the recommendation for everyone. Be especially careful to avoid saturated and trans fats (see page 50), which pose the highest risk of blood fat abnormalities (such as high cholesterol; see page 94), type 2 diabetes, and heart disease. If your child's family history includes abnormal blood fats, type 2 diabetes, or a heart attack before the age of 55, you should reduce his or her fat consumption to these levels at age 2. Follow these guidelines to reduce the fat in your child's diet:

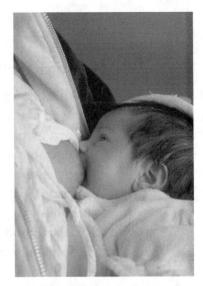

Breast-feeding Is Best

Breast milk is the best source of nutrition during a child's first year of life. Breast milk contains a unique mixture of nutrients, hormones, and proteins essential for digestion, brain development, and growth, and provides antibodies from the mother that ward off infections. Breast-fed babies have fewer digestive problems and food allergies than bottle-fed babies, are less likely to be overweight, and may have a lower risk of developing type 2 diabetes later in life.

- Give fat-free or 1% milk instead of 2% or whole milk.
- Choose the leanest cuts of meat.
- Serve more fish, which contains healthy fats.
- Trim all visible fat from meat and remove the skin from poultry.
- Don't serve butter or stick margarines that contain trans fats; use tub or liquid margarines with plant sterols.
- Bake, broil, grill, poach, or steam foods without added fats instead of frying.
- Serve lower-fat cheeses, such as part-skim mozzarella and low-fat or reduced-fat cheese; although cheese is a good source of calcium, full-fat cheese is high in saturated fat.

- Don't give your child snack foods that contain trans fats such as partially hydrogenated oil. Read food labels for trans fat content.

Watch for Unhealthy Fats

All fats are not the same. The types of fat your child consumes can affect his or her risk of type 2 diabetes and heart disease. So-called good fats—such as polyunsaturated fats and omega-3 fatty acids found in liquid vegetable oils, nuts, and fatty fish such as salmon and mackerel—can keep the arteries healthy and reduce the risk of type 2 diabetes and heart disease. Saturated fats and trans fats, by contrast, can increase the risk. Foods that contain trans fats include stick margarines; many packaged baked goods such as cakes, cookies, and pies; fried foods in fast-food restaurants; and many snack foods such as chips and crackers.

Trans fat grams are now listed on food labels. Read all food labels carefully and resist buying packaged foods that contain trans fats or that list partially hydrogenated vegetable oil in the ingredients list. Two of the foods most loved by children contain trans fats: store-bought cookies and fast-food french fries. Buy only cookies whose labels show 0 grams of trans fats. Purchase frozen french fries that don't contain trans fats so you can bake the fries without added oil at home. Don't use stick margarine or canned shortening when you bake cookies or pie crusts at home. Taking these precautions will protect your entire family from the increased risk of heart disease that trans fats can confer.

On the other hand, some dietary fats are necessary for a child's healthy growth and development. These healthy fats are the monounsaturated and polyunsaturated fats, especially the type of polyunsaturated fats called omega-3 fatty acids. High-quality sources of omega-3 fatty acids are oily fish (such as salmon) and flaxseed. You can also buy eggs that have omega-3 fatty acids added to the yolks. Make sure that the fat your child eats is predominantly from these good fats, while still restricting your child's fat intake to no more than 30 percent of total daily calories. (But don't start limiting the fat intake of your young children until they are 2 years old because babies and toddlers need fat for proper growth and brain development.)

Provide Healthy Lunches

If your child's school provides lunches that are high in fat, salt, and added sugar, pack healthy lunches for your child. Use fiber-rich whole-grain breads and lean meats, poultry, and fish for sandwiches. Buy only reduced-sodium sandwich and deli meats. Spread sandwiches with low-fat condiments such as mustard or low-fat or reduced-fat mayonnaise. Fill the sandwiches with lettuce, tomato, and grilled vegetables. Fortify peanut butter sandwiches with apple butter, banana slices, or raisins or other dried fruit.

Add a packet of baby carrots or celery sticks to your child's lunch bag, and always pack a piece of fresh fruit. To improve the calcium content of your child's lunch, add mozzarella sticks, a cup of low-fat plain yogurt, or a snack-sized container of low-fat yogurt dip for cut-up vegetables. Toss in a small bag of nuts. Leave out the chips, cookies, and snack cakes, which contain a lot of fat, including artery-clogging partially hydrogenated oils (trans fats), which contribute to heart disease risk. Instead, give your child a small bag of pretzels or whole-grain graham crackers (again, always check labels for trans fats and partially hydrogenated oils).

Lactose Intolerance

Some children, especially those of African, Hispanic, Asian, or Native American descent, are unable to digest the sugar lactose that is present in milk and other dairy products. The condition, which is inherited, develops when a child's intestines stop producing an enzyme that digests lactose. The older a child gets, the less tolerant of lactose he or she becomes because production of the enzyme tends to decline with age. Children who have lactose intolerance have abdominal symptoms such as gas, bloating, cramps, or diarrhea shortly after consuming dairy products.

If your child is lactose intolerant, make sure he or she gets enough calcium by serving lactose-free dairy products or calcium-fortified foods such as orange juice or soy milk (make sure these products also contain adequate vitamin D, which helps the body absorb calcium). The calcium added to orange juice (calcium citrate) is especially beneficial because the body absorbs this type of calcium more easily than other types. You can buy lactase enzyme tablets that your child can take before or after eating dairy products, or enzyme drops that you can put into a carton of milk. Calcium supplements are a good way to make sure your child is getting enough calcium; chewable varieties are available for children.

Your child may be able to consume small amounts of milk or cheese at a time without getting an upset stomach. Many people with lactose intolerance are able to tolerate yogurt better than milk because the live bacteria in the yogurt break down the lactose. However, this is not true for commercially frozen yogurt because the manufacturing process kills all of the live bacteria.

A link exists between the consumption of sugary soft drinks and overweight among children, but 60 percent of public and private schools in the United States sell soft drinks during the school day. Soft drink companies often pay for school events or subsidize cash-strapped schools in other ways to get their products into schools. Some schools sign exclusive agreements with the companies to sell only their products. If your child's school sells soft drinks in vending machines or in any other way, become vocal about your opposition to this practice. Get other parents involved so you can present a united front to the school administrators against the policy of selling soft drinks at school.

Shop for Nutrition

As a parent, one of your most important tasks is to shop for healthy foods that you can serve to your growing children. Preparing healthy meals at home requires some advance planning. Before you shop, sit down and decide on your meals for the week. Make a list of the ingredients you will need to provide nutritious, balanced meals. That way, when you need to get dinner on the table quickly, you know what you're going to prepare and the ingredients are already in the kitchen.

Try to avoid buying processed foods and snacks such as cookies and potato chips because they tend to provide lots of calories and harmful fats. Packaged foods also tend to be high in calories, fat, and salt, and are often expensive. Children, especially those who are overweight or who have a family history of high blood pressure, should minimize their intake of salt. Watch for the sodium content on packaged foods and compare labels to find the brands with the least amount of sodium. Packaged items with a low salt content are usually labeled "reduced sodium" or "no salt added."

It can be difficult to figure out exactly how much sugar your child is consuming because sugar can appear on a food label under different names. Table sugar is not the only sweetener added to packaged foods such as cookies and snack cakes; many of these foods contain sugars in the form of sucrose, fructose, maple syrup, molasses, dextrose, sorbitol, and high fructose corn syrup. These sweeteners can dramatically raise the sugar content and calories of foods. To determine how much sugar a packaged food has, check for these sweeteners on the ingredient list. Then look at the Nutrition Facts panel on the food label to see the food's total sugar content; 5 grams of sugar equals 1 teaspoon of granulated sugar.

To help your child adapt to eating less salt and sugar, boost the flavor of meals by using herbs, spices, and lemon and lime juices. Stock up on dried herbs such as basil, oregano, thyme, dill, and rosemary and always keep spices such as cinnamon, nutmeg, paprika, and cumin on hand. When buying garlic powder, onion powder, or chili powder, look for those with no sodium. Seek out fresh herbs in your supermarket or grow some in a sunny window. Offer your child naturally sweet foods such as fruit for snacks and dessert.

Buy fresh foods as often as you can. Focus on fruits and vegetables, low-fat and fat-free dairy products, and lean sources of protein. Go vegetarian one or two nights a week by serving a main course planned around beans, lentils, or tofu. You'll save money, vary your meal routine, and boost your family's fiber intake at the same time.

Avoid arguments with your children over sugary or salty snack foods by not bringing them into the house. Leave the candy, cookies, doughnuts, soft drinks, chips, crackers, and pastries at the store. At snack time, offer your children fresh or dried fruit, cut-up vegetables with a low-fat dip, pretzels, rice cakes, cheese sticks, fat-free yogurt, nuts, or low-fat cottage cheese garnished with fruit. Leftovers from last night's dinner also make good snacks—just watch portion sizes. Serve water or low-fat milk instead of sugary soft drinks when your child is thirsty. Remember that when it comes to your young child's meals and snacks, you are in charge.

Establish Mealtime Routines

Being responsible for your family's meals means that you determine when and what your young children eat. If your overweight child is used to opening up the refrigerator and taking whatever he or she wants whenever, try to break this bad habit now. Children need a mealtime routine as much as they need a bedtime routine. Plan for three meals and two snacks each day. As much as you can, try to establish a daily routine: set times for breakfast, lunch, dinner, and snacks. Most children feel more secure when they know what to expect during the day. When mealtimes are consistent, children get hungry at regular intervals and meals become more relaxed. Serve at least one vegetable or fruit at each meal and include fruits and vegetables at snack time.

Avoid rewarding your children with food or candy for good behavior. Such incentives will get them into the unhealthy habit of rewarding or comforting themselves with high-calorie foods throughout life.

Instead, reward your children with your praise, time, and attention. Give them extra hugs, kisses, and smiles or spend extra time playing a favorite game. After all, your attention is what your child most wants and needs from you.

Get Your Kids into the Kitchen

One easy way to get your children to try new foods is to involve them in meal planning and cooking. Even 3-year-olds can wipe tabletops, tear lettuce, scrub fruits and vegetables, and mix ingredients. They can take pride in making a salad or a side dish, and they gain practical skills when they help you cook. They are also learning about measures, fractions, and even some chemistry and physics. *What makes a pancake turn from liquid to solid? What makes an ice cube melt?* These are just a couple of examples of the interesting discoveries children can make and questions you can answer when you let your children help you cook.

Another benefit is that children are more likely to eat food they participated in preparing. When your children get involved in planning and preparing "good-for-you" foods, they'll want to eat them and

Tips for Picky Eaters

At times, most toddlers and preschool children are fussy about what they do and don't like to eat. Even school-age children can be picky, insisting on eating only certain foods. The good news for parents is that children will usually try new foods if you keep offering them. But never force your children to eat. Serve a variety of foods at each meal and include at least one food that you know your children will eat. Here are some additional tips to help nourish your hard-to-please eaters at home:

- Set a good example by eating nutritious foods yourself. Children copy what their parents do.
- Don't expect your child to like something new the first time you serve it. Serve it again in a week. It usually takes several exposures before children are willing to try a new food.
- Put only a small amount of each food on your child's plate. Let him or her ask for more.
- Let your child touch or smell the new food on his or her plate. It's normal for children to use all of their senses to test out new things.
- To reduce the chances of weight gain, offer only healthy foods. Your child will learn that these are the only foods that are in your home and will eventually eat them.

they're more likely to enjoy them. Having your children help you with meals is also a good way to spend special time with your child, especially after a long day at school. Another benefit is that cooking keeps children away from TV and video games.

Watch Portion Sizes

Kids don't need enormous quantities of food in the years before adolescence. Serve your child food in kid-sized quantities. Doctors recommend serving children 1 tablespoon of each food for every year of age. For example, at dinner, give your 8-year-old about 8 level tablespoons of brown rice and the same amount of applesauce or vegetables, along with a card-deck-sized portion of protein such as poultry. After you measure food portions a few times, you will be able to eyeball the appropriate amounts.

Check the Nutrition Facts labels on all packaged foods that you buy. If the label says there are three servings of peaches in a can, give your child only one-third of the contents. Serve your child his or her dinner on a smaller plate, so it looks like a larger amount of food. When eating out, share an entrée with your child or let two children share one. Never buy huge, 32-ounce sugary soft drinks or slushes for your child—they are sure to pack on the pounds.

Fruit and Vegetable Basics

Fruits and vegetables are essential for good health. Along with whole grains and lean sources of protein, fruits and vegetables should be the foundation of your family's diet. Most people in the United States should at least double the amount of fruits and vegetables they eat every day. Fruits and vegetables are packed with essential vitamins, minerals, fiber, and disease-fighting phytochemicals, which are natural substances in food that work with vitamins, minerals, and fiber to benefit health in many ways.

Because of the high nutrient content of fruits and vegetables, eating plenty of them every day can help reduce your child's risk of the most common chronic diseases—including heart disease, high blood pressure, and some types of cancer—later in life. The abundance of fiber in fruits and vegetables can help protect against insulin resistance and lower the high blood sugar levels that are characteristic of type 2 diabetes.

Best of all, colorful fruits and vegetables look and taste good, so consuming them is easy. Most doctors recommend that children and adults eat 5 to 10 servings of fresh, frozen, or canned fruits (without added sugar) and vegetables every day. A serving can be a medium-sized piece of fruit; ½ cup of fresh, cooked, or canned vegetables or fruit; 1 cup of raw, leafy vegetables; or ¼ cup of dried fruit. Eight ounces of 100 percent vegetable or fruit juice (unsweetened) also count as a serving. Although 100 percent fruit juice is okay once in awhile, you get lots more nutrients from eating a piece of fruit than from drinking fruit juice. Fruit juice is mostly sugar and water, so if your child has a weight problem, eliminating fruit juice is a good way to eliminate extra calories. Just try to make sure that your child doesn't substitute other calorie-dense foods for the fruit juice.

Here's an example of how you can easily fit eight servings of fruit or vegetables into your child's daily routine. For breakfast, serve a sliced orange and top your child's bowl of whole-grain cereal with banana slices or berries. Pack a small salad or carrot or celery sticks in your child's lunch bag along with a piece of fruit, and include a vegetable and a salad at dinner and you've got six servings. Provide cut-up vegetables or fruit as an after-school snack and a second vegetable at dinner and you have effortlessly gotten your child to consume at least two more servings, making a total of eight servings for the day.

Keep fruits and vegetables easily accessible to make them convenient for your child to consume. Buy already-cleaned and cut-up vegetables, such as celery and baby carrots, and keep a bowl of fresh fruit on the counter.

Here are a few more ways to boost your child's consumption of fruits and vegetables:

- Use berries, ripe bananas, and yogurt to make blender smoothies.
- Grill vegetables on your indoor or outdoor grill. Use the leftovers in sandwiches the next day.
- Decorate pancakes and French toast with faces made of raisins, berries, orange slices, and bananas.
- Make guacamole or salsa at home. Use the salsa as a low-fat topping for baked potatoes.
- Serve fruit for snacks and desserts.
- Make frozen-fruit kabobs using pineapple chunks, grapes, and berries.
- Let your child pick out one new vegetable or fruit to try every so often.

- At restaurants, encourage your child to order vegetable-rich dishes such as veggie pizza, pasta with vegetables, or vegetable soup. Take advantage of salad bars. Order coleslaw or a small salad as a side dish instead of fries. Ask for stir-fries and omelets with vegetables. Aim for dishes that make veggies the star and give meat only a supporting role.

Nutrition Concerns for Teenagers

A child's calorie and nutrient requirements soar during adolescence. In addition to more calories, your adolescent will need extra amounts of important vitamins and minerals. Calcium is one mineral that is especially important for rapidly growing teens, both to support fast bone growth and to keep bones strong. Healthy bone development during adolescence can help your child avoid the bone-thinning disease osteoporosis later in life. Your teenager should consume 1,200 milligrams of calcium every day—the equivalent of four 8-ounce glasses of milk.

An adequate amount of vitamin D is also essential for growing teens. Vitamin D helps the body absorb calcium and, because rapid bone growth requires increased vitamin D, it also prevents the softening and weakening of bones. The body is able to manufacture its own vitamin D only when the skin is exposed to the sun's ultraviolet rays. But most children who live in higher latitudes such as the northern United States, where cold weather often forces people to be covered up and to stay indoors, do not get enough vitamin D through sun exposure alone. Many adolescents prefer sedentary indoor activities such as using the computer, playing video games, and watching TV, and they tend to favor sugary soft drinks over vitamin D–fortified milk.

Adolescents also need more B vitamins, found in animal protein, dairy products, and vitamin-fortified foods, to help release energy from the carbohydrates they eat. Many teenagers are deficient in iron, especially teenage girls who are menstruating or are pregnant, teenagers who are vegetarians, and teenage athletes who lose iron during exercise. Good sources of iron include lean red meat, dark meat poultry, pork, iron-fortified breakfast cereals and breads, leafy green vegetables, and dried peas and beans.

It's just as important for teenagers to stay at a healthy weight as it is for younger children. Overweight teenagers have a 70 percent chance of becoming overweight adults. This figure increases to 80 percent if at least one parent is overweight. Being overweight puts your child at risk of a number of serious health problems, including heart disease, type 2 diabetes, high blood pressure, and some types of cancer.

Helping Your Children Get Active

After age 6, children need to get at least 60 minutes of physical activity every day. The exercise does not have to be done all at one time—several 10- or 15-minute periods of activity throughout the day will also work. If your children are not used to being active, encourage them to start with what they can do and gradually build up to 60 minutes a day. Children tend to become less active as they get older. With advances in technology and transportation, many children spend most of their day engaged in sedentary activities, including using a computer, watching TV, and sitting in a classroom. Watching TV for an hour a day increases the risk of obesity by 6 percent, while walking just over half a mile a day decreases the risk by 5 percent. If you both limit your child's TV time and increase his or her time spent being physically active, you can significantly reduce your child's risk of being overweight or, if your child is already overweight, help take off the excess pounds.

Encourage your children to engage in activities or sports they enjoy or would like to learn. Better yet, participate with them. Encourage them to pursue active playtime—going for walks with family members and friends, shooting baskets, or biking or walking to school when they are old enough (and provided you can map out a safe route). Good activities for school-age children are biking, jogging, soccer and other team sports, gymnastics, swimming, skating, and dancing. Try to limit your child's screen time—watching TV, playing video games, or using the computer (unless it's for homework)—to 1 hour or less on weekdays and 2 hours or less on weekends. Not only are such activities sedentary, they also take time away from physical activity, homework, family inter-action, and sleep. Don't allow a TV in your child's bedroom. Watching too much TV may affect a child's ability to achieve academically. In the evening, try keeping the TV off until your children go to bed. This approach is likely to make you more active and productive in the evening as well, and you will probably spend more time engaged with your children.

Children tend to be more active outdoors than indoors. But don't just send your children outside to play—actively play with them. Take them for walks, go to a local playground, and hike and bike with them. When you're at the mall, use the stairs instead of the escalator or elevator. Try new activities. Plant and cultivate a summer garden together and sign up for interesting classes offered by your local park district, community center, or gym. Plan a group or family adventure. Have you ever tried orienteering? It's an outdoor sport long popular in Europe that uses maps to find the way along a path. Many local parks and forest preserves have established permanent paths for both adults and children. You can move through the path at your own pace, form teams to make it a friendly competition, or turn it into a treasure hunt.

Find a convenient exercise time that fits into your child's daily routine, perhaps before or after school or after dinner, when your child will have a harder time finding excuses. Start slowly and gradually build up to more vigorous activities. Begin with 10 minutes and extend the time little by little to 60 minutes a day.

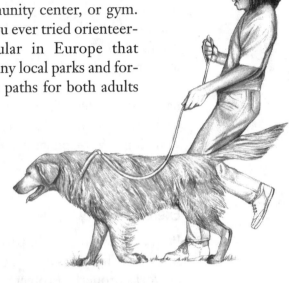

Make Exercise a Daily Routine
Help your child find opportunities to get active on a regular basis. Taking the dog for a daily walk will not only get your child moving, it will also teach him or her responsibility for a pet.

What Type of Exercise Is Best?

To benefit your child, an activity should use the large muscle groups in the legs and arms. But most important, the activity should be fun. Walking, bicycling, swimming, dancing, cross-country skiing, skating, basketball, and soccer are excellent activities for children. Your child should engage in these kinds of activities for 60 minutes most days of the week. The total energy expenditure is more important than the intensity of the activity, so walking 1 mile will burn the same number of calories as running 1 mile. If your child is overweight, he or she may feel more comfortable exercising with other overweight children.

No single sport or activity benefits every child. Try to find activities that your child finds fun and that are appropriate for his or her age and physical ability. Less structured, more flexible lifestyle exercise seems to be better than regimented or high-intensity aerobic exercise for weight control. Children are more likely to become active when they incorporate exercise into their daily routine. Such lifestyle exercise incorporates more physical activity into everyday routines—for example, walking or riding a bike to school instead of getting a ride or taking the stairs instead of an elevator.

Because sedentary activities are such a powerful attraction to so many children, helping your child become more active requires positive reinforcement through a reward system. To encourage increased physical activity, set up an agreement between you and your child that allows him or her to earn points or chips toward rewards that are activity-based, such as going to a museum or the zoo. Every time your child walks the dog or walks a few extra blocks instead of riding in a car, watching TV, or playing a video game, give him or her a few points. After your child earns a preset number of points, reward him or her with a family outing planned around physical activity.

Exercise Safety

If an activity your child participates in requires protective gear, make sure he or she wears it at all times. Check it regularly to make sure it fits or works properly. Protect your child's head by insisting that he or she wear a helmet for activities that can cause head injury, such as riding a bicycle or playing football or baseball. Make sure the helmet is the right size and is tightly buckled so it doesn't slip. Your child needs to keep his or her eyes and ears open while running and playing. Don't let your child wear headphones while exercising outdoors because they can prevent him or her from hearing oncoming cars or people.

When your children are old enough to be outside on their own, make sure you always know where they are going. For walks or bicycle rides, map out a safe route that is familiar to your child and that avoids heavy traffic. Have your child exercise with a friend; having a companion makes activities more fun and can help keep them safe because they can watch out for each other.

Children's smaller size makes them more susceptible than adults to dehydration. Make sure your children drink sufficient amounts of water to stay hydrated, especially when outdoors in hot, humid, sunny weather, of if they sweat heavily. If your child is involved in a prolonged athletic activity, have him or her drink a certain amount of water or a flavored sports drink before, during, and after the activity. Don't wait until your child is thirsty to offer water. Children are less likely to feel thirsty during prolonged play and exercise and they often just don't want to be interrupted. Avoid caffeinated beverages, such as colas and iced tea, because they are dehydrating.

The already increased risk for type 2 diabetes among people in some ethnic groups is raised further when they are not physically active. Many African American and Hispanic American children are less likely than non-Hispanic white children to be involved in organized physical activities such as sports in their neighborhoods. If you live in a neighborhood that lacks safe places to play and exercise, sign up for free or low-cost programs sponsored by your school, church, or park district. If these groups fail to provide options for physical activity for children, talk to community and religious leaders about getting more resources to enable your children to be active and healthy.

Keeping Blood Pressure Normal

Increasing numbers of American children have high blood pressure, which places them at increased risk of developing type 2 diabetes and heart disease. High blood pressure is called a silent killer because it causes no symptoms in the early stages but even so can damage organs and blood vessels. The average blood pressure measurement in American children has risen in recent decades—as many as 1 to 3 percent of children and adolescents may have hypertension or prehypertension (see box on page 238). The increase in the number of overweight children is the major cause of this increase in blood pressure. African American and Hispanic American children usually have higher blood pressure than non-Hispanic white children. Doctors think this difference may result from the higher average weights of children in these groups, but many of these children have probably also inherited a susceptibility to developing high blood pressure that is triggered when they become overweight.

Pediatricians measure the blood pressure of all children ages 3 and older at each well-child visit. Make sure that your child's blood pressure is checked at every doctor visit, especially if your child is significantly overweight or if other members of your family have high blood pressure. If your child has high blood pressure, his or her doctor may recommend an echocardiogram (an ultrasound imaging test of the heart; see page 170) to check for enlargement of the left ventricle (the heart's main pumping chamber). Enlargement of the left ventricle is the most obvious sign of heart damage from high blood pressure in children and adolescents.

The first treatment that doctors recommend for high blood pressure in children is weight loss and exercise. Depending on the degree of hypertension, some doctors may also prescribe an antihypertensive medication such as a diuretic, an angiotensin-converting enzyme (ACE) inhibitor, an angiotensin receptor antagonist, a beta blocker, or a calcium channel blocker.

It's essential to work closely with the doctor to bring your child's blood pressure down to normal to prevent the potential long-term harmful effects of high blood pressure, especially on the heart, blood vessels, and kidneys. Children and teenagers with high blood pressure should never start smoking because smoking can worsen these long-term effects.

How Blood Pressure Is Classified in Children and Teens

Normal blood pressure readings vary depending on a child's gender, age, and height. For this reason, blood pressure readings are given in average percentiles so that children aren't mistakenly diagnosed with high blood pressure if they are taller or shorter than average for their age. Also, normal blood pressure is significantly lower in children and adolescents than it is in adults, so readings that doctors regard as elevated in teenagers can be significantly less than readings considered high in adults.

In children younger than 18, the guidelines define hypertension as blood pressure above the 95th percentile (which means that 95 percent of children of the same gender, age, and height have lower blood pressure). Prehypertension is defined as blood pressure between the 90th and 95th percentiles. In adolescents, prehypertension is defined as blood pressure higher than 120/80.

Stress and the Risk of Type 2 Diabetes

Stress may be another factor that increases the risk of type 2 diabetes in vulnerable children. Researchers have linked stress to insulin resistance (reduced sensitivity of the cells to insulin; see page 12), which can precede type 2 diabetes. The flow of reactions in the body triggered by specific hormones during stressful times can raise blood sugar levels. Foremost among these so-called stress hormones is cortisol, which is produced by the adrenal glands. Normally, cortisol levels return to normal once the stress is dealt with.

However, when stress becomes chronic, cortisol levels remain elevated and can cause fat to accumulate around the abdomen. Fat cells located in the abdomen tend to be less sensitive to insulin than cells in other parts of the body. Some children may have an inherited psychological vulnerability to stress that causes their body to overreact in stressful situations by releasing increased amounts of cortisol. Weight reduction seems to reduce not only insulin resistance in overweight children but also the cortisol level.

Many American children and adolescents are under a lot of stress, from sources including schoolwork, social pressures, expectations to excel, and, perhaps, a part-time job. Getting enough sleep, physical activity, and relaxation can help relieve stress and lower cortisol levels, possibly helping to reduce the risk for type 2 diabetes.

PART SIX

Diabetes during Pregnancy

15

Gestational Diabetes

Each year, nearly 135,000 American women develop type 2 diabetes while they are pregnant, even though their blood sugar levels were normal before pregnancy. This form of type 2 diabetes is known as gestational diabetes. Your risk of having gestational diabetes rises 4 percent for every year of age over 25 you are when you get pregnant; the risk is 60 percent greater at age 40 than at age 25.

Screening for gestational diabetes during pregnancy, diagnosing it early, and effectively treating it as soon as it is diagnosed greatly reduce the risk of complications. Good prenatal care and careful control of blood sugar can make the difference between a healthy, uncomplicated pregnancy and a high-risk pregnancy. Left untreated, gestational diabetes can cause potentially serious problems for the baby and complications for the pregnant woman. Most of the time, gestational diabetes goes away on its own after delivery.

How Gestational Diabetes Develops

During pregnancy, hormones and other substances released from the placenta (the organ that exchanges oxygen and nutrients for waste products between the pregnant woman and the fetus) help the fetus develop.

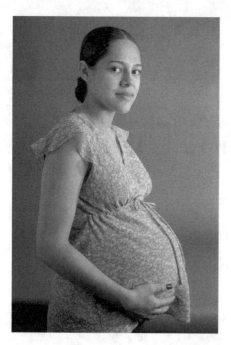

Gestational Diabetes

If you have gestational diabetes, be sure to have frequent prenatal checkups and carefully follow your doctor's recommendations. Maintaining good control of your blood sugar throughout your pregnancy can help ensure a healthy pregnancy and reduce the risk of complications for both you and your baby.

But these same hormones also interfere with the action of insulin (which signals cells to take in glucose from the bloodstream for energy production). These insulin-blocking effects begin to develop in midpregnancy and increase into the third trimester. The pancreas can usually compensate for the insulin-blocking effect by producing more insulin, but if it is unable to manufacture enough insulin, glucose builds up in the blood, resulting in gestational diabetes. The condition usually goes away on its own after pregnancy because the placenta is no longer present to produce the insulin-blocking hormones.

Other factors, some inherited and some related to lifestyle, also seem to play a role. Risk factors for gestational diabetes include being overweight, having a family history of type 2 diabetes (especially a mother who had gestational diabetes), being a member of a high-risk ethnic group (including Hispanic American, African American, Native American, Asian, or Pacific Islander), being over the age of 25, having previously given birth to a baby weighing more than 9 pounds, and having had gestational diabetes during a past pregnancy. You may also be at increased risk if you ever had a stillbirth or a baby born with birth defects.

Every pregnancy is different, and not having had gestational diabetes during a past pregnancy doesn't mean that you won't have it during another. At the same time, having gestational diabetes during one pregnancy does not always mean that you will have it during another. Carefully follow your doctor's recommendations for reducing your risk and make sure you are screened for the disorder during your pregnancy.

Effects of Gestational Diabetes on Women

Most women with gestational diabetes have healthy babies if they control their blood sugar, consume a healthy diet, exercise regularly, and keep their weight gain within the normal range. However, gestational diabetes slightly increases the risk of some problems that could adversely affect a woman's health. The slightly increased risks include preeclampsia, a condition in which blood pressure rises, sometimes to a dangerous level. Gestational diabetes can occasionally also result in preterm (early or premature) labor and can trigger some infections. Having gestational diabetes significantly increases your risk of developing type 2 diabetes later in life. Maintaining good blood sugar control is the most important thing you can do to prevent these problems.

Preeclampsia

A serious condition called preeclampsia can develop in women with gestational diabetes. Preeclampsia usually occurs late in pregnancy and can cause the pregnant woman's blood pressure to soar. Her body also begins to retain excess fluid and to spill protein into the urine. Mild preeclampsia often produces no symptoms, so it is important that you keep all of your prenatal doctor appointments so your doctor can monitor your blood pressure and other vital signs. Symptoms of severe preeclampsia include headaches, blurred vision, sensitivity to bright light, upper abdominal pain, nausea and vomiting, and bloating.

Sometimes preeclampsia progresses to an even more serious condition called eclampsia, in which blood pressure rises so high that it reduces the amount of oxygen that reaches the brain, causing seizures. The seizures can cause a stroke that can be life-threatening to both the pregnant woman and the fetus.

Some overweight women may be mistakenly diagnosed with high blood pressure because the cuff used to measure their blood pressure is too small. If you are significantly overweight, be sure to ask the nurse or the technician who takes your blood pressure if a large-sized cuff was used for the measurement.

If you have mild preeclampsia, your doctor will advise you to get plenty of rest and to eliminate excess salt from your diet to help lower your blood pressure. Severe preeclampsia and eclampsia require hospitalization so you can be given medications to reduce your blood pressure. Your baby may have to be delivered prematurely by inducing labor or by cesarean section if your high blood pressure is preventing the baby from getting sufficient nutrition to grow properly.

Preterm Labor

A normal pregnancy lasts about 40 weeks. Preterm labor refers to the start of labor before the 37th week of pregnancy. The earlier labor begins, the less developed the baby is and the more likely he or she is to have health problems. If this occurs, it places the baby at risk of neonatal jaundice (see page 248) and developmental problems. The incidence of preterm labor in women with gestational diabetes is not very high, but it is somewhat higher than the risk in women who don't have gestational diabetes.

If you think you are going into labor prematurely, call your doctor right away. He or she will probably tell you to go to the hospital, where the staff can evaluate your condition. The doctor may give you medication to help stop labor. In some cases, an evaluation of the amniotic fluid is done to determine if the fetus's lungs have developed sufficiently to function normally after birth. If you deliver prematurely, depending on your baby's condition, he or she will be sent to the nursery or to the neonatal intensive care unit for an evaluation.

Increased Risk of Infection

Gestational diabetes can make a pregnant woman susceptible to developing certain types of infections, particularly urinary tract infections, vaginal infections, and skin infections. High blood sugar levels promote the proliferation of infection-causing microorganisms, especially if blood glucose levels are not well controlled. Bacteria normally present in the urinary tract can multiply rapidly, producing an infection that can spread to the bladder. Symptoms of a urinary tract infection include an urgent need to urinate, a burning sensation during urination, and strong-smelling or bloody urine. If you develop a yeast or urinary tract infection while you are pregnant, drinking a lot of water can help flush out your urinary tract.

A yeast infection is caused by the overgrowth of a fungus called *Candida albicans* that normally grows in the vagina. Women with diabetes are especially susceptible to vaginal yeast infections. To prevent yeast infections, wear cotton underwear and avoid using feminine hygiene sprays or powders, or bubble-bath products. Douching is not recommended at any time because it can promote the development of yeast infections. Symptoms of a vaginal yeast infection include a thick, white, cottage cheese–like vaginal discharge and itching in the vagina. If you think you have a vaginal yeast infection, contact your doctor. Do not treat it on your own with over-the-counter antifungal medications during pregnancy.

The same bacteria and yeast that affect the urinary tract and vagina can also grow on the skin. Overweight women are often affected by yeast infections in the skin folds under the breasts and abdomen. To prevent skin infections, keep your skin clean and dry. If a skin infection occurs during pregnancy, see your doctor.

Effects of Gestational Diabetes on Babies

The risk of gestational diabetes causing serious problems in the fetus is low, and most babies do well unless the gestational diabetes is not controlled. The most important thing you can do to minimize the risks to your fetus once your gestational diabetes is diagnosed is to keep your blood sugar level as close to normal as possible. When problems do occur, the most common are high birth weight, difficult delivery, and a higher risk of delivery by cesarean section. Babies are more likely to have low blood sugar levels and jaundice. Less common problems include the production of too many red blood cells, low calcium and magnesium levels, and damage to the veins in the kidneys. Heart problems and other birth defects are not more common in babies whose mother has gestational diabetes than in babies from normal pregnancies.

High Birth Weight

A baby weighing more than 9 pounds is considered to be larger than normal. Gestational diabetes can increase the chances of having a larger and fatter than normal baby because the excess glucose in the mother's blood overnourishes the fetus, causing the fetus to grow too fast. Overnourishment of the fetus can stimulate the fetus to produce large amounts of insulin, which triggers excess production of fat and causes the organs to become enlarged.

Having a large baby can affect delivery in a number of ways. Very large babies can become injured during natural delivery through the vagina and often must be delivered by cesarean section. If your doctor feels that your fetus is very large or at increased risk of birth injury, cesarean delivery may be recommended. The chances of having a large baby are higher if the baby is overdue. An overdue, or postterm, pregnancy is one that lasts longer than 42 weeks. (The normal length of pregnancy is about 40 weeks.)

Low Blood Sugar

Gestational diabetes sometimes causes a baby to develop hypoglycemia (see page 159), or low blood sugar, after birth. The excess insulin produced by the baby's pancreas in response to high maternal blood sugar can temporarily remain high after birth and cause the infant's blood sugar level to fall. Prolonged low blood sugar can be dangerous for babies because their cells are not getting the fuel they need for growth.

Early and frequent feedings help bring a baby's blood glucose up to a normal level. You will be encouraged to breast-feed. If your baby has hypoglycemia, he or she may be given sugar water or supplemental feedings to raise his or her blood glucose.

Neonatal Jaundice

Babies whose mother had gestational diabetes during pregnancy have a slightly greater risk of having jaundice after birth than babies whose mother did not have gestational diabetes. Jaundice is a condition in which the buildup of a pigment called bilirubin, produced by the normal breakdown of red blood cells, turns the skin and the whites of the eyes slightly yellowish. Jaundice frequently occurs in newborns because they normally have a surplus of red blood cells at birth and, when these cells are broken down, they produce a large amount of bilirubin, which is processed by the liver and excreted in the baby's stool. Because a newborn's liver is not fully developed, it processes bilirubin more slowly than an adult liver, which causes a delay in eliminating the bilirubin that can lead to jaundice.

Babies whose mothers did not have gestational diabetes sometimes have jaundice because all babies have an excess of red blood cells after birth. But babies born to mothers with gestational diabetes tend to have even more red blood cells than usual. The extra red blood cells help stabilize the fetus's oxygen supply, which can be affected by the high insulin levels in the child's bloodstream. The increased red blood cells produce a higher than average chance of developing jaundice.

Immediate and frequent nursing can help reverse jaundice by stimulating bowel movements, which eliminate much of the accumulated bilirubin. Doctors treat abnormally high levels of bilirubin with phototherapy (light therapy), which promotes elimination of the bilirubin in the urine. Light therapy can be done in the hospital or at home. If promptly treated, jaundice is not a serious problem for babies.

Long-Term Effects

The fact that you have gestational diabetes does not mean that your baby will be born with diabetes. But infants born to women with gestational diabetes are at increased risk of developing type 2 diabetes later in life, especially if their mother's blood sugar level was poorly controlled during pregnancy. These children are more frequently overweight and are more likely to have elevated blood pressure than children from normal pregnancies.

Diagnosing Gestational Diabetes

Gestational diabetes rarely causes symptoms, so, to find it, doctors give all pregnant women a glucose screening test. During this test you are asked to quickly drink a sweetened liquid that causes your blood sugar level to rise within 30 to 60 minutes. A blood sample taken from your arm 1 hour later will show how your body processed the sugar. If the test shows that your blood glucose level is elevated, you will be given a more accurate test called an oral glucose tolerance test (see page 91) to determine if you have gestational diabetes.

Doctors give all pregnant women a glucose screening test between the 24th and 28th weeks of pregnancy, because gestational diabetes usually develops by this time. If you are diagnosed with gestational diabetes, you will probably need to have regular tests and more frequent prenatal visits throughout your pregnancy to closely monitor your blood sugar levels and the health of the fetus. For example, you may need to have the A1C test (see page 92), which shows how high your blood glucose has been over the previous 3 months. The higher the amount of glucose in your blood over that period, the higher your A1C test result will be. Your doctor can use this test result to evaluate your baby's health risks.

If your doctor thinks you are at high risk for gestational diabetes, you may be given a glucose tolerance screening test early in pregnancy. High-risk factors your doctor will consider include being over the age of 35, being severely overweight, having a strong family history of type 2 diabetes, or having had gestational diabetes during a previous pregnancy.

Monitoring the Health of the Fetus

If you have been diagnosed with gestational diabetes, your doctor will closely monitor the health of the fetus. This monitoring may include ultrasound or other techniques. One fetal monitoring technique, called the nonstress test, measures the heart rate of the fetus. Normally, when a healthy baby moves, its heart rate goes up. If the heart rate doesn't increase, it can be a sign that the baby could have difficulty during labor. During the test, which usually takes 20 to 60 minutes, two small monitors applied to your abdomen record the fetus's heart rate.

Another monitoring test, called the contraction stress test, evaluates the ability of the fetus to tolerate the low oxygen levels that normally occur during labor contractions. During the test, the doctor stimulates contractions of the uterus (similar to those of labor) by giving you a carefully controlled dose of a medication called oxytocin. If the fetus responds normally—with an increased heart rate—the pregnancy is allowed to continue naturally. If the fetus shows signs of stress—a decreased or abnormal heart rate—the doctor may recommend early delivery. The contraction stress test may be used if the results of the nonstress test are not entirely normal.

Treating Gestational Diabetes

Doctors treat gestational diabetes with a carefully controlled diet designed to keep the pregnant woman's blood sugar level within the normal range for pregnancy (which in all women is lower than nonpregnancy levels). If you have gestational diabetes, your doctor will probably refer you to a dietitian or a diabetes educator who can help you plan meals that will control your blood sugar, taking into account your and your family's food preferences. You will probably be asked to consume three evenly spaced meals a day and one or more snacks between meals or at bedtime. You will be advised to avoid high-fat foods (which can cause excessive weight gain), eat a variety of foods including fruits and vegetables, and watch portion sizes. The number of calories you need depends on how much you weigh and the stage of your pregnancy.

You will have to carefully time your consumption of carbohydrates (starches and grains) so that your body does not take in too much or too little sugar at one time. Your health-care providers will monitor how well your diet is managing your blood sugar and may want to recommend changes every once in a while to get better control over your blood sugar or to meet the needs of your growing fetus.

Exercise can be an important part of managing blood glucose in women with gestational diabetes, as it is in women who have diabetes before they become pregnant. When you contract your muscles during exercise, you increase the transport of glucose into your cells. Physical activity may help you manage gestational diabetes without the need for insulin.

Pregnant women may be more prone to exercise-related injuries if they have been sedentary for a long time. Before recommending an exercise regimen, your doctor will evaluate your personal risk factors and the physical changes you have gone through during your pregnancy, as well as the risk exercise may pose to the fetus and the pregnancy.

> ### WARNING!
>
> ### Exercise during Pregnancy
> Stop exercising and call your doctor immediately if you have any of the following symptoms that persist during or after exercise:
> - Pain in your back, groin, or abdomen
> - Dizziness or feeling faint
> - Shortness of breath
> - Heart palpitations (heartbeats you're aware of) or rapid heartbeat at rest (above 100 beats per minute)
> - Bleeding or fluid loss from the vagina
> - Difficulty walking
> - Contractions of the uterus
> - Absence of fetal movement

If you have not been exercising regularly, start with 30 minutes a day of low-intensity activity such as walking. Non-weight-bearing activities such as stationary cycling, swimming, and doing arm exercises are also good choices. Rest for half an hour after exercising. The risks of low-intensity exercise during pregnancy are minimal, even for women who were sedentary before their pregnancy.

Your doctor will test your blood sugar level regularly. He or she will probably also ask you to monitor your blood sugar yourself at home (see page 126) at least four times a day to determine if your eating and exercise routines are maintaining your blood sugar within the desired range. If your diet and exercise regimens fail to adequately control your blood sugar, you may need to give yourself insulin injections two to four times a day throughout the rest of your pregnancy. Your doctor may need to adjust your insulin dose periodically, depending on how well your blood sugar is controlled. (Taking insulin during your pregnancy will not affect the fetus or the pregnancy because the hormone does not cross the placenta.)

Some doctors are prescribing oral medications instead of insulin to women whose diet and exercise regimens have not kept blood sugar in the desirable range. If your doctor prescribes an oral diabetes medication, your blood sugar will be monitored just as closely as it would be if you were taking insulin.

After delivery, your blood glucose level will probably return to normal right away. Your blood glucose will be monitored in the hospital after delivery to make sure that it has returned to normal. However, your having gestational diabetes puts you at risk of developing type 2 diabetes later in life. Your risk of developing type 2 diabetes within five years of your pregnancy is 40 to 50 percent, and your lifetime risk is 70 to 80 percent. The likelihood of developing type 2 diabetes after having gestational diabetes is especially high if don't lose the weight you gained during pregnancy or if you become heavier. Your doctor will want to screen you for the disorder two months after delivery and at every future physical examination to make sure your blood sugar stays in the healthy range. Reducing your weight, changing to a healthy diet, and exercising more can help you avoid type 2 diabetes in the future.

Glossary

This glossary defines some common medical terms you'll find in this book. Italicized words within definitions are words that are defined elsewhere in the glossary.

A1C test   A test that gives a picture of a person's average blood glucose level over the past 3 months. It shows how well a person's treatment for diabetes is working over time. Blood sugar attaches to the *hemoglobin* in red blood cells, forming a substance called hemoglobin A1C. The A1C test measures the percentage of this combined substance.

acanthosis nigricans   A skin disorder, most often occurring in young people who are obese and have very high blood insulin levels. The condition produces raised, brown patches on the neck, armpits, and groin. It is strongly linked to an increased risk of type 2 diabetes. Losing weight helps the patches disappear.

ACE inhibitors   A class of medications prescribed for *high blood pressure* and heart failure that block an enzyme (angiotensin-converting enzyme or ACE) that causes arteries in the kidneys to constrict and the kidneys to retain salt.

adrenal glands   A pair of small, triangular glands located directly above the kidneys. They make and release *hormones* that affect nearly every system in the body. Stress hormones such as adrenaline and cortisol increase *blood sugar levels*.

adult-onset diabetes   The term formerly used to refer to type 2 diabetes, before the disorder began to appear in children.

aerobic exercise   Physical exercise that requires the heart and lungs to work harder to meet the muscle's increased demand for oxygen. Examples of aerobic exercise include brisk walking, jogging, biking, stair climbing, and cross-country skiing.

alpha cells   A type of cell inside the *islet cells* of the *pancreas* that produces *glucagon*, a *hormone* that raises the level of blood sugar.

alpha-glucosidase inhibitors   A class of medications prescribed for diabetes that are known as starch blockers, because they slow the digestion of starches in food. Examples are acarbohydrateose and miglitol.

antibodies   *Proteins* in blood and tissue fluids that protect the body from invading foreign organisms such as bacteria, viruses, and harmful toxins. Antibodies are part of the body's *immune system*.

antioxidants   Vitamins, minerals, and other substances in the body that protect against cell damage caused by excess amounts of molecules called *free radicals*, normal by-products of the body's *metabolism*. Free radicals are also produced when *blood sugar levels* are high.

artery   A blood vessel that carries oxygen-filled blood away from the heart to supply the rest of the body.

atherosclerosis   The buildup of hardened fatty deposits called plaque inside *artery* walls. Atherosclerosis can narrow the blood vessels, reducing or blocking blood flow and increasing the risk of a *heart attack* or a *stroke*.

autoimmune disorder   A disorder in which the *immune system* mistakenly produces *antibodies* that attack the body's own cells and tissues. Type 1 diabetes is an autoimmune disorder in which antibodies attack the *beta cells* of the *pancreas*.

beta cell   A type of cell inside the *islet cells* of the *pancreas* that produces the *hormone insulin*. In type 2 diabetes, the beta cells increase insulin production, but eventually cannot keep up with the demand and begin to fail, reducing the body's ability to make insulin.

biguanides   A class of medications prescribed for *diabetes* that reduce the amount of sugar made by the *liver*. An example is the medication *metformin*.

blood glucose monitoring, self   The measurement of blood *glucose* levels by a person with diabetes using a fingerprick drop of blood, a strip, and a *glucose meter*.

blood pressure   The force that blood exerts against the walls of the *arteries* as it is pumped through the body by the heart. It is measured with a machine that produces two numbers: the upper, higher number is *systolic* pressure and the lower number is *diastolic* pressure. A blood pressure reading of 120/80 is considered normal for adults.

blood sugar   A form of sugar known as *glucose* that circulates in the blood and is one of the main fuels for the body's cells. After *carbohydrate* is broken down into glucose, it can be converted into energy or stored. Abnormally high levels of glucose in the blood signify the presence of diabetes.

blood sugar level   Also known as the blood *glucose* level. The concentration of the sugar glucose in the blood, as determined by a laboratory or home blood test. Blood sugar levels are elevated in people with uncontrolled diabetes.

C-reactive proteins   Proteins present in the blood that indicate *inflammation*. In some cases, high levels may indicate an increased risk for heart disease.

calcium   A mineral that is essential for strong bones and teeth. It also plays a role in muscle contraction (including the heart), blood clotting, and nerve function. Dietary sources include dairy products, canned salmon and sardines with their bones, and leafy green vegetables.

calcium channel blockers   A group of medications used to treat *high blood pressure*. They cause blood vessels to relax by keeping calcium out of them.

calorie   A unit of measurement representing the amount of energy contained in food. Eating too many calories can cause weight gain if the extra calories are not burned through physical activity.

carbohydrate   One of three main categories of food nutrients. (The others are *protein* and *fat*.) A category of food that includes sugars, *starches*, and *fiber*, which are broken down by the body to form the sugar glucose. Management of *blood sugar levels* in people with diabetes depends on the careful control of carbohydrate consumption.

carbohydrate counting A system of managing food intake to regulate *blood sugar levels* that tracks the grams of carbohydrates consumed at all meals and snacks.

cardiovascular system Also called the circulatory system. The network, formed by the heart and blood vessels, that pumps blood and transports it to organs and tissues throughout the body.

cholesterol A type of *fat*, or *lipid*, made by the liver that the body needs to help produce *hormones* and bile (a fluid that aids the digestion process). Cholesterol is also absorbed into the bloodstream from cholesterol-rich foods. Cholesterol is part of the outer lining (membrane) of cells. The two main types of blood cholesterol are high-density lipoprotein (*HDL*, the good cholesterol) and low-density lipoprotein (*LDL*, the bad cholesterol).

chromium An essential mineral that helps the body make a glucose tolerance factor, which helps insulin function better. Chromium levels are low in people in some parts of the world but not typically in the United States. Chromium is being studied for the treatment of diabetes because some studies have found that chromium supplements may improve *blood sugar* control.

coma A state of unconsciousness. A coma can result from a too high or too low level of sugar in the bloodstream, among other causes. Diabetic coma refers to an extreme form of high blood sugar that causes *ketoacidosis* and unconsciousness.

complications Harmful effects of diabetes. They can be acute, short-term effects, such as *hypoglycemia*, or chronic, long-term effects, such as damage to nerves and blood vessels, kidney damage, and blindness.

continuous blood glucose monitoring A system that records *blood sugar levels* at frequent intervals to identify patterns in sugar levels over time. Continuous monitoring of blood sugar can give a doctor information that can help him or her adjust treatment but is not intended to replace *fingerstick testing*.

dehydration A potentially dangerous reduction in the amount of water in the body. Symptoms include increased thirst, dry mouth and tongue, nausea, and fatigue.

diabetes   A condition in which too much *glucose* is present in the blood. There are two main forms: *type 1 diabetes* and *type 2 diabetes*. *Gestational diabetes* develops during pregnancy and is usually related to type 2 diabetes. A more rare type, diabetes insipidus, occurs as the result of a deficiency of a *hormone* released by the pituitary gland in the brain; diabetes insipidus is not linked to the level of blood glucose.

diabetic coma   See *coma*.

diabetic retinopathy   See *retinopathy, diabetic*.

diastolic blood pressure   The second, lower number in a *blood pressure* reading, which indicates the amount of pressure in the blood vessels when the heart rests between beats and fills with blood.

dietary cholesterol   The kind of *cholesterol* found in animal foods such as dairy products, meat, and eggs. It is one source of blood cholesterol.

dietary exchange system   A method devised to help people with diabetes plan meals to gain better control over their blood *glucose* level. The system divides food into three major groups: *carbohydrates*, meat and meat substitutes, and *fats*. Each group contains foods that are similar in *calorie*, carbohydrate, *protein*, and fat content, which makes them interchangeable.

fasting plasma glucose test   Sometimes called a fasting blood sugar test because it's given after a person has fasted for at least 8 hours. A test that measures the level of sugar in the blood, plasma (the liquid component of blood), or serum (the sticky liquid left in the blood after the solid parts have clumped). The fasting plasma glucose test is a reliable way to diagnose *diabetes*. Levels at 99 mg/dL or below are normal; 100 to 125 mg/dL indicate *impaired fasting glucose* (a form of *prediabetes*); higher than 125 mg/dL can indicate a diagnosis of diabetes.

fat   One of three main categories of food nutrients. The others are *protein* and *carbohydrates*. There are many different types of dietary fat: *saturated, monounsaturated, polyunsaturated, dietary cholesterol, omega-3 fatty acids*, and *trans fats*. High amounts of saturated fat and trans fats in the diet raise the risk of heart disease.

fatty acids   A basic unit of blood fats. When not enough of the sugar *glucose* is available to the cells, the body burns fatty acids for energy.

By-products of this process are *ketones*, which cause the acid level in the blood to rise too high. A buildup of ketones in the body can produce a life-threatening condition called *ketoacidosis*, which can cause dangerous irregularities in many organs of the body, including the heart.

fiber   An indigestible nutrient found in fruits and vegetables that passes through the digestive tract without being absorbed. Fiber provides bulk to keep the digestive tract working properly. There are two types of fiber: soluble and insoluble. Consuming foods containing soluble fiber can help keep *blood sugar levels* normal and can reduce the risk of heart disease.

fingerstick glucose test   A test used to determine how much of the sugar glucose is present in the blood. A small drop of blood from the fingertip is placed on a disposable test strip, which is coated with chemicals that blend with the glucose in blood. The strip is placed in a glucose meter, which measures how much glucose is present.

folic acid   A B *vitamin* essential for cell growth and repair and for the production of red blood cells. Consuming adequate amounts of folic acid may reduce levels of homocysteine, a chemical that indicates the presence of chronic *inflammation* in the blood vessels and possibly an increased risk of heart disease. During pregnancy, consuming sufficient folic acid helps protect against birth defects affecting the brain and the spine.

free radicals   Also called oxygen free radicals. *Molecules* produced in the body through normal cell activity or from external factors such as radiation or cigarette smoke. In excessive amounts, free radicals damage or destroy cells—a major cause of disease and aging.

fructose   A form of sugar, found in fruit and honey, that is sweeter than table sugar and is used to sweeten many foods, including soft drinks. It is converted into glucose by the liver.

gestational diabetes   A form of *diabetes* that develops during pregnancy because the placenta produces *hormones* and other factors that block the effects of the hormone *insulin*. The condition usually resolves on its own after delivery, but the risk of developing diabetes later in life is very high.

glucagon   A *hormone* released by the *pancreas* that raises the level of sugar in the blood. When blood *glucose* levels fall below normal, glucagon instructs the *liver* to break down stored sugar (*glycogen*) and send it into the bloodstream to prevent *hypoglycemia*. Glucagon can be injected to raise blood sugar levels quickly; home glucagon kits are available to people with diabetes for such emergencies.

glucose   A simple sugar that is one of the main sources of energy for the body's cells. Also known as dextrose. Food in the diet is broken down into glucose (for use by the cells) or is stored as *glycogen*.

glucose meter   A small, battery-powered device used by people with diabetes to measure the amount of sugar in a small sample of blood taken from the tip of a finger. This test is commonly known as a *fingerstick test*.

glycemic index   A system that rates the blood sugar response of the body to a particular food, compared with its reaction to a standard amount of *glucose*. The glycemic index rates *carbohydrate* foods by their effects on blood sugar. Carbohydrates that break down rapidly in the bloodstream have a high glycemic index; those that break down more slowly have a lower glycemic index.

glycogen   Sugar that is stored in the body. The body stores extra *glucose* as glycogen in the *liver* and muscles. When *blood sugar levels* begin to fall, the liver releases stored glycogen into the bloodstream.

HDL cholesterol   High-density lipoprotein *cholesterol*. A type of cholesterol made in the *liver* and carried in the blood. Also called the good cholesterol, it protects against heart disease by helping to clear *LDL cholesterol* from blood vessels.

heart attack   Also called myocardial infarction. Sudden damage to a section of the heart muscle from lack of blood, usually as a result of a blockage of blood flow in one of the coronary arteries by a blood clot.

hemoglobin   The *protein* in red blood cells that carries oxygen to the cells.

high blood pressure   Also called hypertension. A condition in which blood pressure is consistently elevated. High blood pressure is common in people with *type 2 diabetes* and is a risk factor for heart disease.

high-density lipoprotein (HDL) cholesterol   See *HDL cholesterol*.

hormones   Chemical messengers that are produced by a network of glands called the endocrine system. Hormones are released directly into the bloodstream, which carries them to target organs and tissues throughout the body, where they perform specific functions. The hormone *insulin* is needed for *glucose* to enter the cells, which use it for energy or store it.

hydrogenated fats   See *trans fats*.

hyperglycemia   Abnormally high levels of *glucose* in the blood.

hypertension   See *high blood pressure*.

hypoglycemia   Abnormally low levels of *glucose* in the blood. Hypoglycemia can occur when people with diabetes take their diabetes medication or insulin but fail to eat enough or at the right time, increase their physical activity, take too much medication or insulin, or drink too much alcohol.

immune system   A system in the body responsible for fighting disease. Its main function is to identify foreign substances such as bacteria, viruses, or parasites and then launch a defense against them. This defense is known as the immune response. One way it functions is by producing *proteins* called *antibodies* to eliminate foreign microorganisms that invade the body.

impaired fasting glucose   A form of *prediabetes*.

impaired glucose tolerance   A form of *prediabetes*.

inflammation   Redness, swelling, heat, and pain in a tissue caused by injury, infection, or hypersensitivity to an allergen

insulin   A *hormone* produced by the *pancreas* that enables the body's cells to use the sugar *glucose*. In people with *type 2 diabetes*, the pancreas does not make enough insulin to get glucose into the cells, causing glucose to build up in the bloodstream.

insulin-dependent diabetes   See *type 1 diabetes*.

insulin resistance   A condition in which the cells are insensitive to the effects of *insulin*, making it more difficult for them to take in and use or store the sugar *glucose*. Can eventually lead to *type 2 diabetes* if the *pancreas* cannot make enough insulin to keep blood glucose at a healthy level.

insulin resistance syndrome   Also called *metabolic syndrome* and *syndrome X*. A group of conditions strongly associated with each other and with an increased risk of *cardiovascular disease*. These conditions include obesity (especially when concentrated around the abdomen), *prediabetes* or *type 2 diabetes*, elevated levels of *triglycerides* in the blood, low levels of good *HDL cholesterol* in the blood, *high blood pressure*, and *polycystic ovarian syndrome*.

iron A *mineral* that is essential for the production of many enzymes (*proteins* that speed the rate of biological reactions) and for the formation of *hemoglobin*.

islet cell Also called an *islet of Langerhans* cell. A cell in the *pancreas* that produces *hormones* such as *insulin* or *glucagon* that are released into the bloodstream. These hormones regulate the level of the sugar *glucose* in the bloodstream.

islet cell transplantation An experimental procedure in which clusters of cells called *islet cells* are taken from a donor *pancreas* and transferred into the *liver* of a person with *diabetes*. Once implanted, the *beta cells* in these islets start to make and release *insulin*. Now performed only in people with *type 1 diabetes*.

islets of Langerhans Clusters of cells in the *pancreas* that produce *hormones* such as *insulin* and *glucagon* that regulate blood sugar.

juvenile diabetes Another name for *type 1 diabetes*, which usually first appears during childhood or adolescence.

ketoacidosis The buildup of high levels of *ketones* in the blood. Common symptoms include excessive thirst, nausea and vomiting, rapid heartbeat, abdominal pain, drowsiness, and a fruity odor to the breath. A characteristic pattern of deep, rapid breathing punctuated by deep sighs (known medically as Kussmaul breathing) is a sign of the condition. Diabetic ketoacidosis is a medical emergency that without immediate treatment can progress to seizures, coma, and death.

ketones Chemicals that the body makes when it has to break down *fat* to produce energy. Insufficient *insulin* is one reason the body makes a large amount of ketones. Ketones accumulate in the blood and then overflow into the urine. They can injure cells. They impart a fruity odor to the breath.

LDL cholesterol Low-density lipoprotein *cholesterol*. A harmful type of cholesterol made by the *liver* and transported in the blood; it can cause fatty deposits to build up in artery walls, leading to heart disease. Hereditary factors and eating foods that are high in *saturated fat* (such as fatty meats, butter, and whole-milk dairy products) and *trans fats* (such as stick margarine) increase blood levels of LDL.

lipids   Fats that are present in the body. Some fats are used for energy. Examples of lipids are *cholesterol, fatty acids,* and *triglycerides.*

lipoprotein   Substances made of *lipids* and *protein.* Many fats, including cholesterol, are carried in the blood in the form of lipoproteins.

liver   An organ located in the upper right part of the abdomen that performs many vital functions. It secretes the digestive juice bile and processes *protein, carbohydrate,* and *fat.* It detoxifies poisons, breaks down worn-out red blood cells, manufactures *cholesterol,* and converts excess blood sugar to stored fat and *glycogen.*

low-density lipoprotein (LDL) cholesterol   See *LDL cholesterol.*

magnesium   An essential mineral that plays several important roles in the body, including the transmission of nerve signals. It also helps produce energy from food, assists in normal muscle control, regulates the heartbeat, and helps make protein. Dietary sources include vegetables (especially dark-green leafy vegetables), soy products, legumes and seeds, nuts, and whole grains.

meglitinides and D-phenylalanine derivatives   A class of medications prescribed for diabetes that help the *pancreas* make more insulin. An example is repaglinide.

metabolic syndrome   See *insulin resistance.*

metabolism   The physical and chemical processes that occur in a living organism. Also a term that describes the way cells chemically use fuel from food to keep the body functioning.

metformin   A medication prescribed for *type 2 diabetes* that reduces the amount of *glucose* made by the *liver.*

monounsaturated fat   A type of fat found in olive, peanut, and canola oils that lowers harmful *LDL cholesterol* and raises beneficial *HDL cholesterol.*

myocardial infarction   See *heart attack.*

obesity   A condition in which a person weighs 20 percent or more over the maximum desirable weight or has a BMI of 30 or higher. Children are considered obese if their BMI falls above the 95th percentile for their age. Obesity is the primary factor contributing to the development of *type 2 diabetes*.

omega-3 fatty acids   A type of *polyunsaturated fat* that promotes heart health by lowering *inflammation*, inhibiting blood clotting, and widening blood vessels. Good dietary sources of omega-3 fatty acids are oily fish such as salmon and tuna, and flaxseed.

oral glucose tolerance test   A test used to diagnose *diabetes* by comparing *blood sugar levels* before and after drinking a liquid containing *glucose* dissolved in water.

oxidation   A chemical reaction in cells that converts food into energy. High rates of oxidation can produce an excess of *free radicals*, which can damage cells.

oxygen free radicals   See *free radicals*.

pancreas   A gland located behind the lower part of the stomach that produces the *hormone insulin* and secretes digestive juices into the intestine through ducts. In *type 1 diabetes*, an immune system dysfunction causes damage to and breakdown of the *beta cells* in the pancreas, stopping them from generating enough insulin to keep *blood sugar levels* normal. In *type 2 diabetes*, blood sugar is elevated because the beta cells cannot make enough insulin to overcome the insensitivity of the cells to insulin.

pancreas transplant   A surgical procedure in which the *pancreas* of a person with diabetes is replaced with all or part of a healthy pancreas from a donor. Pancreas transplants are sometimes used for people with *type 1 diabetes*, but remain experimental for those with *type 2 diabetes*.

partially hydrogenated oils   See *trans fats*.

plaque, arterial   Also called atheroma. A patch of fatty buildup in an *artery* wall that can reduce blood flow or cause obstruction by a blood clot.

polycystic ovarian syndrome   A condition characterized by elevated levels of male hormones (androgens), the presence of numerous small cysts in the ovary, the accumulation of fat around the abdomen, irregular menstrual cycles, failure to ovulate, and excess facial hair. The condition is strongly linked to the presence of *insulin resistance* and is associated with a high risk of developing *type 2 diabetes*.

polyunsaturated fat   A type of dietary *fat* (found in corn, sunflower, safflower, sesame, flaxseed, and soybean oils) that reduces total *cholesterol* levels but may also lower beneficial *HDL cholesterol.*

potassium   An essential mineral that helps the body maintain water balance, conduct nerve signals, contract muscles, and maintain a normal heartbeat.

prediabetes   A condition characterized by a *blood sugar level* that is elevated but not high enough to indicate a diagnosis of *type 2 diabetes.* Without treatment, prediabetes is likely to lead to type 2 diabetes.

protein   A category of food that is used by cells for growth and repair. Dietary sources include meat, fish, poultry, dairy products, nuts, and dried beans.

puberty   The body's natural transition from physical and sexual immaturity to maturity, characterized by the maturing of the sexual organs, development of secondary sexual characteristics and reproductive functions, and growth spurts.

retinopathy, diabetic   Damage to the retina, the light-sensitive membrane at the back of the eye, from *diabetes.* Is the single most common cause of irreversible blindness in industrialized countries.

salt-sensitive   Describes a person whose *blood pressure* goes up or down in relation to the amount of *sodium* in his or her diet.

saturated fat   A type of dietary *fat* (found in meat, dairy products, and coconut and palm oils) that contributes to a higher level of *LDL cholesterol* in the blood, which is thought to increase the risk of *heart attack* and *stroke.*

sodium   Also known as table salt. An essential mineral that helps the body maintain water balance and *blood pressure.*

starch   A type of *carbohydrate* in plant foods such as cereal, bread, pasta, grains, and rice. Is also found in some fruits such as bananas and vegetables such as potatoes.

stem cells   Primitive cells present in embryos or in the bone marrow of adults that can grow into many different kinds of cells. Researchers are looking at ways to coax stem cells into becoming the *beta cells* in the *pancreas* that produce *insulin.* This process could lead to a cure for *type 1 diabetes* because the newly grown beta cells could become a replaceable source of cells for *islet cell transplantation.*

strength-training exercises Also known as resistance training. Repeated bouts of intense activity done with free weights or circuit-type weight machines that forces the body's muscles to work against an outside weight. Exercises such as sit-ups, pull-ups, push-ups, and leg lifts are also considered strength-training conditioning because they set the muscles against the weight of the body. Strength training can help control *blood sugar levels*.

stroke Blocked blood circulation to the brain that causes brain cells to die from the resulting lack of oxygen. Nearly 80 percent of strokes are caused by blockage from a blood clot; 20 percent result from a ruptured blood vessel that bleeds into the brain.

systolic blood pressure The first, or higher, number in a *blood pressure* reading indicating the pressure in the blood vessels when the chambers of the heart contract and pump blood through the *arteries*.

sulfonylureas A class of medications for *diabetes* that stimulate the *pancreas* to release more *insulin* into the bloodstream, effectively lowering *blood sugar levels*. Examples include glyburide, glimepiride, and glipizide.

thiazolidinediones A class of medications prescribed for *diabetes* known as *insulin* sensitizers because they make the body's cells more sensitive to insulin's effects. Examples are pioglitazone and rosiglitazone.

trans fats Also called *hydrogenated fats* and *partially hydrogenated fats*. Fats that are made during the manufacturing of stick margarine and canned shortening and used in many processed, baked, and deep-fried foods such as snack cakes, cookies, and doughnuts. Trans fats contribute to higher levels of both total *cholesterol* and harmful *LDL cholesterol* in the blood.

transplant Transfer of an organ or tissue from one part of the body to another or from one person to another. See *pancreas transplant*.

triglycerides One of the major types of *fat* that circulates in the blood. A high level in the blood can indicate an increased risk of heart disease, *high blood pressure*, and *type 2 diabetes*.

type 1 diabetes Formerly known as *insulin-dependent diabetes* and *juvenile diabetes*. An *autoimmune disorder* that develops more frequently during childhood and adolescence than in adulthood. People with type 1 diabetes usually need injections of the *hormone insulin* to stay alive. The disorder is much less common than *type 2 diabetes*.

type 2 diabetes   Formerly known as *non-insulin-dependent diabetes* and *adult-onset diabetes*. A disorder in which the body has difficulty using *insulin* to control the level of *glucose* in the blood. Being overweight is a major cause. Once found only in middle-aged people, type 2 diabetes is now occurring in increasing numbers of children and young adults. People with type 2 diabetes can often control their *blood sugar levels* with weight loss, exercise, and diet, but some need to take sugar-lowering medication or daily *insulin* injections.

unsaturated fat   A type of fat that tends to be soft or liquid at room temperature. Lowers the risk of heart disease and *stroke*. Eating *polyunsaturated fat* instead of *saturated fat* reduces harmful *LDL cholesterol* but may also lower beneficial *HDL cholesterol*. *Monounsaturated fats* reduce LDL cholesterol and raise HDL.

vein   A blood vessel that carries oxygen-depleted blood back from organs and tissues to the heart to get a fresh supply of oxygen.

very low-density lipoprotein cholesterol   See *VLDL cholesterol*.

vitamin   A chemical present in food that is essential for normal functioning of the body. Except for vitamin D, which the skin produces when it is exposed to sunlight, vitamins are not manufactured by the body and must be consumed from food.

VLDL cholesterol   Very low-density lipoprotein. A fat made by the liver and transported in the blood. VLDL carries cholesterol in the blood. A high VLDL cholesterol level increases the risk of heart disease.

Index

abdominal area, fat concentrated in, 9, 13, 20, 27, 29, 33, 34, 53, 98, 129, 197, 238

abdominal curl (exercise), 73

acanthosis nigricans, 14, 181, 199, 207, 208

ACE inhibitors, 174, 186, 238

Achilles-tendon problems, 82

A1C test, 92–93, 249–250

acupuncture, 147

adolescents. *See* children and young adults

adrenal glands, 6, 238

adrenaline, 6, 27, 128, 177

adult-onset diabetes. *See* type 2 diabetes

aerobic exercise, 71–72, 251
  See also exercise

African Americans, 94, 202, 208, 237, 244

age (aging), 20–21
  children and young adults. *See* children and young adults
  Dietary Guidelines for Americans, 117
  fitness and, 79
  gestational diabetes and, 244

as risk factor, 1, 5, 7, 13, 20–21

air travel, special precautions for, 152–153

alcohol consumption, 23, 53, 61–62, 94, 95, 116–117, 138, 179, 221
  hypoglycemia and, 160

alpha-glucosidase inhibitors, 132, 133

alternative and complementary therapies, 146–149

American Diabetes Association, 112

American Dietetic Association, 112

amputation, 5, 178, 179

anaphylaxis, 138

androgens, 6, 29

angina, 124, 127, 168

angiogram, coronary, 171, 176

angioplasty
  balloon, 172, 174, 176–177
  laser, 172

angiotensin receptor antagonists, 238

antioxidants, 58–60, 65, 67

arterial plaque, 166, 172, 175

Asian Americans, 202–203, 208, 244

aspirin, 168, 169

atherectomy, 172

type 1 diabetes and, 7
type 2 diabetes and, 21–22,
    197–198, 200–201, 208
weight and genetics, 98
family relationships, 219
fast foods, 23–24, 60, 197, 212
fasting insulin test, 209
fasting plasma glucose test, 15,
    90–91, 209
fatigue, 9, 89
fats, 112, 116
    blood cholesterol and, 50–54
    in child's diet, 225–226
    counting fat grams, 40
    in a healthy diet, 46, 49–54, 108,
        225
    monounsaturated, 38, 49, 50, 52,
        226
    plant sterols, 49, 52
    polyunsaturated, 38, 49, 50, 52,
        226
    saturated. *See* saturated fats
    stocking the pantry, 63–64
    trans fats. *See* trans fats
    weight loss and limiting, 38–39
feet
    common problems, 125, 179
    daily foot checks, 179–180
    footwear for exercising, 76, 80,
        82–83, 125
    fungal infections, 181
    nerve damage, 177–178
    tips for keeping them healthy,
        179–180
    ulcers, 178, 179, 180
fiber, 42–43, 46, 47–49, 110–111, 231
    medications affected by high-fiber
        diet, 111
    water-insoluble, 48, 110
    water-soluble, 48, 110–111
fingerstick glucose test, 139–140,
    214–215
fish, 64
flexibility exercises, 74–75
    See also exercise

folic acid, 57, 168
Food and Drug Administration
    (FDA), 146–147, 216
food labels, reading, 25, 39, 51, 52,
    66, 68, 121, 226
food preparation, 46, 117
food substitutions, 65, 219
footwear for exercising, 76, 80,
    82–83, 125
free radicals, 58
French fries, 203
fruits, 46, 49, 63–64, 204, 213, 225,
    229, 231–233
    carbohydrates from, 110
    daily servings of, 109, 231–232
    Dietary Guidelines for Americans,
        59, 116
    fiber in, 111
    phytochemicals in, 59
fungal infections, 181

gangrene, 178, 179
genetics. *See* family history
gestational diabetes, 28–29, 92,
    243–252
    causes of, 243–244
    child's risk of developing type 2
        diabetes and, 198, 205–206, 249
    diagnosing and treating, 249–252
    effects on babies, 247–249
    effects on women, 244–247
    ethnicity and, 202
    monitoring the health of the fetus,
        250
    recovery after pregnancy, 244, 252
    as risk factor for type 2 diabetes,
        245, 252
    risk factors for, 244
gingivitis, 188–189
gingko biloba, 148–149
ginseng, 148
glaucoma, 184–185
glossary, 253–266
glucagon, 6, 8, 9
    emergency kit, 160

inhaled, 138–139
injections, 6, 135–138, 215–216, 217, 218, 252
intensive treatment, 139, 154
manufacture of human, to treat diabetes, 10
production of, by the pancreas, 6, 8, 9, 10
programming non-beta cells to produce, 145
role of, 5, 8, 9
side effects of, 137–138
types of, 135
insulin C-peptide test, 209
insulin pens, 136–137
insulin pumps, 137
insulin resistance, 5, 11–12, 12–14, 27, 33, 98–99, 196, 231
causes of, 12–13, 238
consequences of, 13–14
during puberty, 206
insulin resistance syndrome, 16
insulin sensitivity, 11, 12, 47, 69
gestational diabetes and, 244
intensive insulin treatment, 139, 154
intertrigo, 199
iron, 57, 58, 233
iron-deficiency anemia, 58
ischemia, 169
islet cell transplants, 144–145

jaundice, neonatal, 246, 247, 248–249
jet injections (of insulin), 137
jock itch, 181
joint problems, 199, 209

ketoacidosis, diabetic, 10, 135, 141, 163–164
ketone bodies, 10
kidney dialysis, 187
kidney disease, 5, 9, 174, 186–187, 195
Kussmaul breathing, 163

lactic acidosis, 216, 221
lactose intolerance, 204, 227
laser angioplasty, 172
leg lift/leg extension, 79
legumes, 111
lifestyle factors. *See* alcohol consumption; exercise; nutrition; smoking
lithium, 111
low birth weight, 198, 206
low blood sugar. *See* hypoglycemia
low-density lipoprotein (LDL) cholesterol, 24, 47, 53, 95–96, 111, 167, 174
fats and, 50–54
lunch
providing healthy, 226–228
school lunches, 197, 226
lycopene, 59, 67

magnesium, 57, 61, 148
malabsorptive surgery for weight loss, 103, 104, 105
margarine, 38, 51
massage, 129
meal planning, 107–109, 213–214
involving children in, 230–231
mealtime routines, 229–230
meats, 64, 112
medical identification bracelet or necklace, 151
medications
blood pressure, 94, 174–175, 190, 238
cholesterol, 54, 96, 111, 167
for diabetes, 6, 69, 131–141, 215–217
for erection problems, 190–191
for heart disease, 171–172
high-fiber diet and, 111
for peripheral neuropathy, 178
during pregnancy, 154, 252
for preterm labor, 246
questions to ask about, 134

medications (*continued*)
  side effects of, 133–134, 137–138, 139, 190, 216
  for stroke, 175
  weight loss, 101–102
meditation, 101, 129
meglitinides, 132, 134, 137
menopause, 13, 94, 95
menstruation, irregular, 29
metabolism, 17, 98
metformin, 69, 132, 134, 215, 216, 221
microalbumin, 186
mindfulness exercises, 101
minerals, 55, 57, 61
  antioxidants, 58
  in fruits and vegetables, 49
miscarriage, 154
monounsaturated fats, 38, 49, 50, 52, 226
MRI (magnetic resonance imaging), 176
muscle weakness, 178

National Heart, Lung, and Blood Institute, 119
Native Americans, 21, 201–202, 208, 244
necrobiosis lipoidica diabeticorum, 181–182
neonatal jaundice, 246, 247, 248–249
nerve damage, 5, 177–179, 195
  symptoms of, 177–178
neurological evaluation, 124
non-insulin-dependent diabetes. *See* type 2 diabetes
nonstress test (fetal monitoring), 250
nutrition, 45–68, 107–122, 166
  calories. *See* calories
  carbohydrate counting, 114–115
  dietary exchange system, 112–113
  Dietary Guidelines for Americans, 59–60, 116–117, 213
  for family, 62–68, 211–214
  food substitutions, 65, 219
  gestational diabetes and, 250–251
  glycemic index, 115, 118
  guidelines, 108
  healthy diet, components of a, 45–46
  poor diet as risk factor, 7, 21, 22, 23, 203–204
  prevention of type 2 diabetes, 15, 224–234
  weight loss and. *See* weight loss
  See also specific nutrients, e.g. carbohydrates; fats; protein
nuts, 64, 67

obesity or being overweight, 1, 7, 13, 16, 17–18, 19–20, 94, 95, 98–99
  body mass index (BMI), 20, 34–35, 200
  children and young adults, 196, 198–200, 208, 222–223, 233–234
  gender and, 17
  gestational diabetes and, 244–245
oils, vegetable, 38, 50–52
  stocking the pantry, 64
olive oil, 50, 52, 65
omega-3 fatty acids, 15, 49, 52, 226
omega-6 fatty acids, 49
ophthalmologists, 183, 185
oral glucose tolerance test, 15, 91–92, 209, 249, 250
orlistat, 102
osteoporosis, 70, 71, 233
ovaries, 6
  polycystic. *See* polycystic ovarian syndrome
overweight, being. *See* obesity or being overweight

Pacific Islander descent, people of, 208, 244
pancreas
  beta cells, 7, 10, 12, 20, 145
  functions of, 6, 8, 9, 10
  gestational diabetes and, 244

programming non-beta cells to produce insulin, 145
pancreas transplants, 144
pantry, stocking the, 63–67, 228–229
parathyroid glands, 6
perimenopause, 98
periodontal disease, 30, 188–190
peripheral artery disease, 176–177
peripheral neuropathy, 177–179
phentermine, 102
phototherapy (light therapy) for neonatal jaundice, 249
physical examinations, 17
   before becoming pregnant, 154
   before starting exercise program, 75–76, 78, 123–125, 251
physical inactivity. *See* sedentary lifestyle
phytochemicals, 59
picky eaters, tips for, 230
Pilates, 74
Pimas, diabetes among the, 21, 201
pituitary gland, 6
placenta, 243, 244, 252
polycystic ovarian syndrome, 14, 16, 29, 207–208, 209
polyunsaturated fats, 38, 49, 50, 52, 226
portion sizes, 39, 43, 59–60, 119, 197, 231
potassium, 57, 61
poultry, 56–57, 64
prediabetes, 14–17, 28
   statistics, 1
preeclampsia, 245
pregnancy
   alcohol consumption during, 62
   diabetics who become pregnant, 153–155
   Dietary Guidelines for Americans, 117
   exercise during, 251
   gestational diabetes. *See* gestational diabetes
   insulin resistance and, 13

insulin sensitivity and, 11
   overdue, or postterm, 248
premature births, 154, 206, 245, 246
preterm labor, 246
prevention of type 2 diabetes, 33–69
   in children and young adults, 223–239
   diet and. *See* nutrition
   exercise. *See* exercise
   weight, maintaining a healthy. *See* weight loss
processed and refined foods, 22, 23–25, 47, 60, 120–121, 197, 204, 228
progesterone, 6
protein, 37–38, 64, 204
   in a healthy diet, 46, 54–55, 108
   high-protein diets, 36
   kidney disease and, 187
psyllium, 111
puberty, insulin resistance during, 206, 208
pump-up (exercise), 79
push-up, modified, 73

radiation therapy (bracyhtherapy), 172
refined foods. *See* processed and refined foods
relaxation techniques, 147
restrictive surgery for weight loss, 103, 104, 105
retinal detachment, 124, 125
retinal hemorrhage, 125
retinopathy, diabetic, 124–125, 126, 154, 183–184, 185
rewarding children, appropriately, 229–230, 236
RICE for exercise-induced injuries, 81
ringworm, 181
risk factors, 19–30
   age, 1, 5, 7, 13, 20–21
   for children and young adults, 197–206

risk factors (*continued*)
    dietary, 7, 21, 22, 23, 203–204
    ethnicity. *See* ethnicity
    family history. *See* family history
    for gestational diabetes, 244
    obesity. *See* obesity or being over-
      weight
    pregnancy. *See* gestational diabetes;
      pregnancy
    sedentary lifestyle. *See* sedentary
      lifestyle
    sleep, lack of, 27–28
    smoking. *See* smoking
    stress. *See* stress

salt (sodium), 23, 25, 46, 57, 60–61,
    109, 116, 120–122, 225, 228, 245
    DASH diet, 99, 119–122
    foods high in, 60–61
    high blood pressure and, 25, 60–61
saturated fats, 23, 24, 36, 38, 40, 45,
    46, 49, 50, 52, 53, 54, 67, 95, 109,
    225, 226
school lunches, 197, 226
    providing healthy, 226–228
sedentary lifestyle
    of children, 196
    exercise. *See* exercise
    as risk factor, 1, 7, 13, 21, 22, 23,
      25–26, 204–205
seizures, 162, 163, 245
serving sizes, 39, 43, 59–60
shoes for exercising, 76, 80, 82–83,
    125
sibutramine, 102
sickness, special care of diabetes dur-
    ing a, 149–151
side effects of medications, 133–134,
    137–38, 139, 190, 216
side stretch, 75
sildenafil, 190
skin problems, 180–182, 199,
    246–247
    acanthosis nigricans, 14, 181, 199,
      207, 208

    fungal infections, 181
    tip for avoiding, 182
skipping meals, 43, 108
sleep, 27–28, 168
sleep apnea, 209
smoking, 23, 26–27, 94, 139, 175,
    177, 179, 189, 221, 238
    stopping, 167–168
snacks, nutritious, 67–68, 213
    timing of, 108
sodium. *See* salt (sodium)
soft drinks, sugary, 23, 24–25, 46,
    203, 212, 225, 228, 229, 231
sores that don't heal, 90
spices, 64, 229
statins, 96
stem-cell research, 145–146
stent, 172, 176–177
stillbirths, 154, 244
strength-building exercises, 72–74,
    79, 126–127
    See also exercise
stress, 27, 94, 238–239
    managing, 27, 128–129, 168
    while sick, 150
stress test, exercise, 124, 170
stroke, 9, 14, 23, 26, 166, 173–175
    preventing, 174–175
    test, 175
    treating, 174
    warning signs, 173–174
sugar, 23, 24–25, 64, 228–229
    in a healthy diet, 46, 109
    in soft drinks. *See* soft drinks,
      sugary
sulfonylureas, 132, 133, 137
surgery
    for heart disease, 172
    weight loss, 103–105, 213
symptoms
    of type 1 diabetes, 7
    of type 2 diabetes, 8, 9, 87–90
syringes, insulin, 136

tadalafil, 191

target heart rate, 77
teenagers. *See* children and young adults
teeth, caring for your, 188
testicles, 6
testing for diabetes, 15–16, 90–96, 208, 209
  gestational diabetes, 249–250
testosterone, 6, 29, 207
thallium exercise stress test, 170
thiazolidinediones, 132, 134
thirst, 9, 88, 222
"thrifty genes," 22–23
thrush, 181
thyroid gland, 6
thyroxine, 6
tPA (tissue plasminogen activator), 175
traffic-light diet (for kids), 211
trans fats, 23, 24, 38, 39, 46, 51–52, 53, 67, 68, 95, 109, 203, 225, 226, 227
transplants
  islet cell, 144–145
  kidney, 187
  pancreas, 144
traveling, special care when, 151–153
treatment
  of heart disease, 171–172
  of stroke, 174
  of type 1 diabetes, 7, 10
  of type 2 diabetes, 6, 69, 131–141, 209–223
triceps press, 73
triglycerides, 14, 20, 23, 53, 95, 96, 166, 167
  prediabetes and, 16
triiodothyronine, 6
TV watching, 26, 212, 224, 231, 234
type 1 diabetes, 1, 5–7, 10, 195
type 2 diabetes
  in children. *See* children and young adults
  complications. *See* complications

diagnosis, 90–96, 206–207, 208–209
early stages of, 8–9, 11–12, 14–17
overview, 5–6, 8–9
prevention. *See* prevention of type 2 diabetes
risk factors. *See* risk factors
statistics, 1, 17, 20
symptoms of, 8, 9
treatment, 6, 69, 131–141, 209–223

ultrasound, 176, 250
urinary tract infections, 178, 246
urination, frequent, 9, 88, 222, 246

vaginal yeast infections, 181, 246–247
vanadium, 148
vardenafil, 190
vegetables, 46, 49, 56–57, 63, 204, 213, 225, 229, 231–233
  carbohydrates from, 110
  daily servings of, 109, 231–232
  Dietary Guidelines for Americans, 59–60, 116–117
  phytochemicals in, 59
vegetarians, 54
vitamin A, 56
vitamin B complex, 56–57, 168, 233
vitamin C, 56
vitamin D, 56, 95, 233
vitamin E, 56
vitamin K, 56
vitamins, 55–57
  antioxidants, 58
  fat-soluble, 49, 56
  in fruits and vegetables, 49
  losing weight and, 37
  water-soluble, 56–57

waist measurements, 20, 34
water, 48, 229
  exercising and, 76, 80, 127, 236–237